QBASE RADIOLOGY: 2

MCQs FOR THE FRCR

QBASE RADIOLOGY: 2
MCQs FOR THE FRCR

By

Dr. R. R. Misra BSc(Hons), MBBS, FRCS, FRCR
Specialist Registrar in Radiology
St Mary's Hospital
London

Dr M. C. Uthappa BSc, MBBS, FRCS, FRCR
Specialist Registrar in Radiology
St Mary's Hospital
London

Dr P. S. Richards MB ChB, MRCP, FRCR
Senior Registrar in Radiology
Royal London Hospital
Whitechapel
London

Dr D. Evans BSc(Hons), MBBS
Specialist Registrar in Radiology
Royal London Hospital
Whitechapel
London

Dr O. Chan MBBS, FRCS, FRCR
Consultant Radiologist
Royal London Hospital
Whitechapel
London

QBASE RADIOLOGY: 2

MCQs FOR THE FRCR

QBase series developed and edited by

Edward J. Hammond MA BM BCh MRCP FRCA
Specialist Registrar
Department of Anaesthesia
Southampton General Hospital

Andrew K. McIndoe MB ChB FRCA
Consultant Anaesthetist
Sir Humphry Davy Department of Anaesthesia
Bristol Royal Infirmary

© 2001
Greenwich Medical Media Ltd.
137 Euston Road
London
NW1 2AA

ISBN 1 84110 040 4

First Published 2001

Apart from any fair dealing for the purposes of research or private study, or criticism or review, as permitted under the UK Copyright Designs and Patents Act, 1988, this publication may not be reproduced, stored, or transmitted, in any form or by any means, without the prior permission in writing of the publishers, or in the case of reprographic reproduction only in accordance with the terms of the licences issued by the Copyright Licensing Agency in the UK, or in accordance with the terms of the licences issued by the appropriate Reproduction Rights Organization outside the UK. Enquiries concerning reproduction outside the terms stated here should be sent to the publishers at the London address printed above.

The right of R.R. Misra, M.C. Uthappa, P.S. Richards, D. Evans and O. Chan to be identified as authors of this Work has been asserted by them in accordance with the Copyright, Designs and Patents Act 1988.

The publisher makes no representation, express or implied, with regard to the accuracy of the information contained in this book and cannot accept any legal responsibility or liability for any errors or omissions that may be made.

A catalogue record for this book is available from the British Library

Produced and Designed by
Saxon Graphics Limited, Derby

Printed in the UK by
Ashford Colour Press Ltd

CONTENTS

Exam 1	1
Answers	15
Exam 2	27
Answers	41
Exam 3	55
Answers	69
Exam 4	83
Answers	97
Exam 5	109
Answers	123
Exam 6	137
Answers	151
Exam 7	165
Answers	179

QBase Radiology on CD-ROM

CD-ROM System Requirements & Installation Instructions 192

Dedicated to my late father, Dr. K. C. Misra.

RRM

Dedicated to my late brother, Maj. M. C. Muthanna.

MCU

Preface

The MCQ exams contained within this book have been structured to conform to the exact format of the Part I FRCR examination, and as such we recommend that the candidate attempt each examination within a two hour time period.

In addition the authors have, where relevant, tried to give full explanations to their answers in an attempt to provide a useful *aide memoire* for the candidate.

R.R.M.
M.C.U.
P.S.R.
D.E.
O.C.
London
May 2000

Editor's note

Notes for users of QBase FRCR on CD-ROM

Please read carefully and print the HELPFILE on the QBase CD-ROM

QBase is an interactive MCQ examination program designed to help candidates improve their performance in negatively marked MCQs. Please follow the installation instructions at the printed in back of the book. The QBase program resides on your hard disk and reads the data from whatever QBase CD is in your CD drive. If you install QBase from this CD, it will update previous version of the program. Owners of previous QBase titles will then have all the new functions available to them. All QBase CDs will work with the new program. To check for successful installation of the new program, check the Quick Start Menu screen. It should have 6 exam buttons. Not all QBase titles will use this button. We encourage you to print and read the Helpfile.rtf on the CD-ROM. It contains more detailed information on the features and analysis functions in QBase.

QBase FRCR 2 contains 420 questions in Physics, Anatomy, and Techniques. The 'Autoset an Exam' option on this CD will present you with exams containing 60 questions made up as follows; Physics 20, Anatomy 20, Techniques 20. The 7 predefined exams on this CD are constructed in the same way and are exactly the same as the ones printed in the book. **Please note that there are only 6 exam buttons on the Quick Start Menu screen**. To access Exam 7 you must go to the Main Menu screen and select the 'Resit exam' option. From the dialogue box that appears, select the 'exam' directory of the **QBase CD** in your **CD drive** and then the exam you wish to attempt. You can generate your own customised exams using the "Create your own exam" option. You can save completed exams and your responses to your hard disk allowing you to review or resit the same paper at a later stage in your revision. Please refer to the helpfile for more information. To further enhance your revision, instead of selecting the 'Resit exam' button, we suggest you select the 'Resit shuffled exam' button. The leaves within each question will be randomly shuffled, removing your ability to remember the pattern of the answers rather than the facts. The exam analysis functions in QBase will provide you with a detailed breakdown of your performance.

We hope that you will find these notes, suggestions and improvements in the program useful in your preparation for the exam. Don't be discouraged if you only achieve a low overall score at first. The MCQ paper is perceived as a threatening test of breadth of knowledge and most candidates fear negative marking. Whilst not a substitute for knowledge and proper preparation, QBase will assist you in assessing your exam technique and provide feedback that will lead to improved performance.

Good luck!

Edward Hammond
Andrew McIndoe

QBase Series Developers/Editors
May 2000

Exam 1

QUESTION 1

Regarding radioactivity

A. The unit of radioactivity is the becquerel (Bq) where 1 Bq is 1 disintegration per second
B. The concentration of radioactivity is measured in Bq/Kg
C. At a temperature of absolute zero the radioactive decay process is unaffected
D. In stable heavy nuclei, there are an excess number of neutrons relative to the number of protons
E. X-rays have a greater maximum possible energy than gamma rays

QUESTION 2

Regarding the filtration of x-rays

A. Tissue contrast is increased
B. The photoelectric effect predominates
C. A beryllium window results in less attenuation of the beam compared to a glass window
D. When aluminium is being used as a filter facing an anode, a backing filter is also required
E. For undercouch fluoroscopy, 2.5 - 4 mms of aluminium is the recommended added tube filtration

QUESTION 3

Dosimetry

A. A thimble chamber has an atomic number (Z) approximately equal to that of air
B. An exposure rate meter requires a resistor in parallel to a voltmeter
C. In an exposure meter, the outer wall of an ionization chamber is connected to the capacitor
D. The response of an ionization chamber increases with increasing wall thickness
E. The use of a lead cylinder cathode in a Geiger-Muller tube, increases the detection of efficiency of gamma rays

QUESTION 4

Concerning x-ray film

A. The supercoat consists of a thin later of polyester
B. Film speed is a reciprocal of the exposure needed to produce a density of 1 above base plus fog
C. Exposing a film to bright light after fixation will destroy the image of the film
D. Fog is more noticeable at low densities
E. Incomplete washing of the film following fixation will result in the film developing a brown layer of silver sulphide

QUESTION 5

In a rotating anode tube, the x-ray tube assembly is primarily immersed in oil for the following reasons

A. To provide lubrication for the rotating anode
B. To filter the x-ray beam
C. To assist in the cooling of the anode following an exposure
D. To provide electrical insulation
E. To provide mechanical protection to the x-ray tube assembly

QUESTION 6

Radiation Protection

A. The relative biological effectiveness (RBE) of radiation is the ratio of the number grays of two radiation qualities which give the same biological effect on the same material in the same time
B. The RBE for x-rays is 10
C. The annual whole body dose limit for a radiation worker is ten times greater than that for a member of the public
D. Natural background radiation contributes 5 mSv to the annual whole body dose per person in the UK
E. The largest contributor to natural background radiation is radon and thoron

QUESTION 7

The following are true

A. The gamma of a film refers to the maximum slope of the shoulder region of the characteristic curve
B. High gamma films have a narrow exposure latitude
C. Low gamma films have a narrow exposure latitude
D. Low gamma films have low inherent film contrast
E. The optical density of a film plotted against the reciprocal of the exposure given to that film is known as the characteristic curve

QUESTION 8

Regarding film processing

A. Films are washed with water prior to fixing
B. The developer is kept alkaline to keep the pH between 9.6 - 10.6
C. Glutaraldehyde in the developer acts as an anti fogging agent
D. The purpose of the fixer is to immediately stop any further development of latent image centres
E. The fixer contains aluminium salts which harden the film and reduce drying time

QUESTION 9

Regarding the resolution of an image intensifier

- A. The centre of the image intensifier screen has a brighter image than the periphery
- B. The periphery of an image intensifier screen has a better resolution than the central field
- C. There is less geometric distortion at the periphery of the intensifier screen compared to the centre
- D. The effects of geometric distortion are more pronounced in small field intensifiers
- E. Electrons at the periphery of the intensifier field are less accurately focused than those at the centre and produce unequal magnification

QUESTION 10

Concerning the effects of ultrasound

- A. Heat is produced when ultrasound interacts with tissue
- B. Cavitation is seen in the lung
- C. There is no correlation between the intensity of the ultrasound beam used and the chance of biological effects
- D. Diagnostic ultrasound intensities are safe
- E. Ultrasound does not cause ionization

QUESTION 11

Regarding the interaction of x-rays or gamma rays with tissue

- A. Produce secondary electrons
- B. Are more for higher atomic number materials
- C. At lower energies, the interaction occurs in a manner which is predominantly inversely proportional to the square of their energy
- D. Scatter predominantly in a forward direction
- E. The interaction may occur with either free or bound electrons

QUESTION 12

In diagnostic radiology

- A. Dental tubes usually have rotating anodes
- B. Fine and coarse focus are selected by the application of a different current to a single filament
- C. In linear tomography the greater the angle of swing the thicker the cut
- D. When multiple simultaneous tomographic cuts are made, all the film screen combinations have the same sensitivity
- E. Rotating anode tubes do not need to be filled with oil

QUESTION 13
Before a radiofrequency pulse if applied to a patient within a MR scanner magnet

A. Each of the patients hydrogen nuclei is precessing about an axis which is parallel to the field of the magnet
B. There are equal numbers of hydrogen nuclei in a spin-up and spin-down positions
C. Within each slice being imaged, there is a net magnetic vector parallel to the static magnetic field
D. Within each slice being imaged, there is a net magnetic vector in a plane perpendicular to the static magnetic field
E. A signal is not be detected

QUESTION 14
Scatter radiation

A. Reducing the field area reduces scatter production
B. Applying compression reduces scatter production
C. Use of a grid increases the amount of scatter reaching the film screen combination
D. Use of an air-gap technique decreases the amount of scatter reaching the film due to absorption of photons within the air gap
E. Use of a lower kV produces more forward scatter

QUESTION 15
Regarding intensifying screens

A. Film screen combinations are more sensitive to x-ray exposure than film alone
B. The use of screens reduces patient dose
C. The use of screens reduces exposure times and consequently decreases movement unsharpness
D. The use of screens reduces tube loading
E. The use of screens increases film gamma

QUESTION 16
Mammography

A. In mammography, a molybdenum filter is used primarily to remove the characteristic radiation produced at a molybdenum anode
B. A single rare earth front screen is usually used
C. For macro-radiography, a focal spot size of 0.1mm is used
D. Compression of the breast only serves to cause discomfort to the patient
E. Films with a gamma of about 3 are used

QUESTION 17
Regarding dose limits

A. The annual whole body dose limit for members of staff over 18 years of age is 50 mSv
B. The annual whole body dose limit for members of the public or visitors is 15 mSv
C. The annual dose limit to the eyes for a trainee aged 16-18 years is 45 mSv
D. The annual dose limit to the extremity for a member of staff over 18 years of age is 500 mSv
E. Staff are designated as classified if they exceed 20% of any annual dose limit

QUESTION 18
Regarding ultrasound

A. Coarse gain regulates the height of echoes from all depths
B. Increasing the near gain control enhances near echoes
C. Increasing the far gain control is used to enhance all distant echoes
D. Increasing the intensity control to a transducer produces stronger echoes at all levels
E. Reject control discriminates against echoes from a particular depth

QUESTION 19
Regarding spatial encoding in MRI

A. The application of a Z field gradient (gradient along the axis of the static magnetic field) in slice selection, occurs simultaneously with a 90 degree radio frequency pulse
B. Slice thickness may be increased by increasing the Z field gradient
C. Slice thickness may be reduced by decreasing the radio frequency band width
D. The application of the frequency encoding gradient occurs when the MR echo signal is being received
E. Field of view may be increased by increasing the receiver band width

QUESTION 20
The following statements regarding MRI sequences are true

A. Gradient echo sequences (GES): Time for repetition (TR) = 500 ms and time to echo (TE) = 25 ms, flip angle = 40 degrees: T1 weighting
B. GES: TR = 250 ms, TE = 10 ms, flip angle = 5 degrees: proton density weighting
C. GES: TR = 50 ms, TE = 5 ms, flip angle = 70 degrees: T1 weighting
D. GES cannot be used for volume acquisition of data
E. In GES, scanning is fast enough to allow data acquisition during a single breath hold

QUESTION 21

Regarding the mandible

A. The symphysis menti fuses by adolescence
B. Most of the permanent dentition calcify by three years of age
C. The first permanent molar erupts by six months in majority
D. During arthrography of temporomandibular joint both upper and lower synovial spaces can be visualised by one injection into either space
E. The mental foramen lies between the pre molars

QUESTION 22

Regarding the venous drainage of the leg

A. The small saphenous vein pierces deep fascia to enter the popliteal vein in the popliteal fossa
B. The long saphenous vein enters the femoral vein just proximal to the inguinal ligament
C. The long saphenous vein has no valves above the knee
D. Paired venae comitantes accompany the three main arteries in the calf
E. The profunda femoris vein joins the femoral vein posteriorly 4-12 cm below the inguinal ligament

QUESTION 23

Regarding blood supply to the lower limb

A. The popliteal artery ends as it passes under the fibrous arch of soleus muscle
B. Popliteus tendon separates the popliteal artery from the posterior surface of the femur
C. The anterior tibial artery crosses the ankle joint midway between the malleoli
D. The posterior tibial artery can be palpated anterior to the medial malleolus
E. The calcaneal artery is a branch of the peroneal artery

QUESTION 24

At the shoulder

A. The joint capsule is attached to the surgical neck of the humerus
B. The subacromial bursa communicates with the shoulder joint
C. The tendon of the long head of biceps lies within the joint
D. The humeral epiphysis is wholly intracapsular
E. Deltoid causes flexion of the arm

QUESTION 25

The following statements are true

A. Humeral supracondylar fossae are more common in females
B. The carpal angle normally measures 150-170 degrees
C. The radial collateral ligament is attached to the annular ligament
D. A sesamoid bone is seen at the thumb interphalangeal joint in 10% of cases
E. A notch may be seen on the medial aspect of the distal radius of a child

QUESTION 26

The following statements are true

A. The internal pudendal artery leaves the pelvis via the lesser sciatic foramen
B. The superior gluteal artery arises from the posterior division of the internal iliac artery
C. The superior rectal artery is a branch of the internal iliac artery
D. The common iliac artery bifurcates at the pelvic brim
E. The round ligament is supplied by the uterine artery

QUESTION 27

The vagina

A. Measures approx. 20 cm in length
B. Has a blood supply from vaginal and uterine arteries
C. Has a transverse lumen for most of its length
D. Has a deep anterior and shallow posterior fornix
E. In its upper two thirds drains to external and internal iliac nodes

QUESTION 28

The coeliac artery

A. Is the artery of the embryonic mid gut
B. Has a branch supplying the oesophagus
C. Gives off the right gastric artery
D. Arises from the abdominal aorta behind the median arcuate ligament
E. Supplies the third part of the duodenum

QUESTION 29

Regarding the liver

A. The bare area lies to the right of the inferior vena cava
B. The quadrate lobe is functionally part of the left lobe
C. The porta hepatis is enclosed between two layers of lesser omentum
D. It is supplied entirely by the superior mesenteric artery in 2.5% of cases
E. Has hepatic veins which are entirely intrahepatic

QUESTION 30

Regarding the kidneys

A. The left kidney may normally be up to 17 cm in length
B. The kidneys may move as much as 5 cm with respiration
C. Pelvic kidneys take blood supply from external iliac artery
D. The renal pelvis usually lies anterior to the renal artery at the hilum
E. The renal vein lies anterior to the renal artery at the hilum

QUESTION 31

The following statements are true

A. Lymphoid follicles in the rectum may measure up to 6 mm normally
B. The post rectal space may measure up to 2 cm at S4 level
C. The lesser and greater sacs communicate through the epiploic foramen
D. The gastroduodenal artery passes anterior to the neck of the pancreas
E. The portal vein lies posterior to the epiploic foramen

QUESTION 32

The following are true about ligaments of the vertebral column

A. The anterior longitudinal ligament extends from the basilar part of the occipital bone to the upper sacrum
B. The posterior longitudinal ligament is firmly attached to the intervertebral discs
C. The supraspinous ligament is replaced as the ligamentum nuchae above the 4th thoracic vertebra
D. The ligamentum flavum passes from posterior surface of one lamina to the anterior surface of the lamina below
E. In CT and MRI the ligamentum flavum appears thicker in successively lower axial slices

QUESTION 33

The following statements are true

A. The left main bronchus is 2cm long and 1.2cm wide
B. The anterior relation of left main bronchus is the pulmonary trunk
C. The posterior relation of left main bronchus are oesophagus and IVC to its right
D. One of the superior relations of left main bronchus is the pulmonary artery
E. The lingula lobe bronchus comes off the lower lobe bronchus and has superior and inferior divisions

QUESTION 34

The following statements are true

A. The left subclavian artery arises at the level of T3/4 disc space
B. The scalenus posterior muscle divides subclavian artery into 3 parts
C. The first part of subclavian artery lies posterior to the lung apex
D. The subclavian artery and vein are separated by the 3 scalenus muscles on each side
E. The subclavian artery becomes the axillary artery at the lateral border of the first rib

QUESTION 35

The following statements are true

A. The external carotid artery divides into its terminal branches within the parotid gland
B. The parotid gland is divided into superficial and deep portions with relation to the course of facial nerve
C. There are normally 24 deciduous teeth
D. The first molar is the first permanent dentition to erupt
E. The parotid duct pierces the masseter muscle

QUESTION 36

Regarding the fourth ventricle

- A. It is the cavity of mid and hind brain
- B. The cavity is heart shaped when viewed from behind
- C. The roof of the cavity superiorly is formed by the superior medullary velum
- D. The inferior medullary velum lies between the superior cerebellar peduncles
- E. It has two medial and two lateral openings to communicate with the subarchnoid spaces

QUESTION 37

Tributaries of the internal jugular vein are

- A. Inferior petrosal sinus
- B. Branches of the pharyngeal plexus of veins
- C. Facial vein
- D. Maxillary vein
- E. Superior and inferior thyroid veins

QUESTION 38

The following statements are true

- A. The anterior fontanelle closes by about 18 months after birth
- B. The posterior fontanelle closes by about 12 months after birth
- C. The supraorbital foramen lies at the junction of medial third and lateral two thirds of the supraorbital margin
- D. The zygomatic arch is formed by temporal and zygomatic bones
- E. The pterion is 3.5cm behind and 1.5cm above the frontozygomatic suture

QUESTION 39

The hypothalamus includes the following

- A. Infundibular stalk
- B. Optic chiasm
- C. Posterior perforated substance
- D. Mamillary bodies
- E. Tuber cinereum

QUESTION 40

With respect to thoracic vertebrae

- A. From level T3 the bodies become larger from above downwards
- B. The body is heart shaped
- C. Articulation with the corresponding rib is at the upper costal demifacet
- D. The pedicle arises from the upper part of the body
- E. The superior articular process projects upwards from the junction of the pedicle and lamina

QUESTION 41

Regarding mammography

A. Compression allows the use of a higher kVp
B. With a non-grid film-screen system and a Molybdenum target, 16-20 kVp gives the highest soft tissue contrast
C. Double emulsion film is usually used
D. Soft tissue contrast depends on a high ratio of photoelectric effect to Compton absorption
E. A rhodium target and rhodium filter can be used for dense breasts

QUESTION 42

When imaging the parathyroid glands

A. 201 Tl is trapped by the normal thyroid
B. 201 Tl is trapped by the hyperactive parathyroid glands
C. 99mTc-pertechnetate is trapped by the normal thyroid
D. 99mTc-pertechnetate is trapped by the normal parathyroid glands
E. 99mTc-MIBI is trapped by normal thyroid but not normal parathyroid tissue

QUESTION 43

During sialography the following projections are appropriate

A. Parotid : Lateral oblique with 15-20 degrees cephalad tube angulation
B. Submandibular : Oblique lateral with a 20 degree cephalad tube angulation
C. Submandibular : True lateral
D. Parotid : Occlusal
E. Parotid : True PA

QUESTION 44

Regarding renal ultrasound

A. An ectopic kidney is more common on the left than the right
B. The incidence of horseshoe kidneys is 1/400
C. Renal agenesis is more common than renal ectopia
D. Renal agenesis is more common on the right
E. Bladder volume is calculated by the product of the three planes x 0.5

QUESTION 45

Regarding the intravenous pyelogram

A. Calyceal detail is better demonstrated on ultrasound
B. An inferior venacaval filter is a contraindication to compression
C. The maximum nephrogram density is dependent on the peak plasma level of contrast media, the glomerulo-filtration rate, and the rate of resorbtion of sodium and water in the proximal convulated tubule
D. Low osmolar contrast media produces greater pelvicalyceal distention than high osmolar contrast media
E. The peak nephrogram phase occurs slightly later with low osmolar

contrast media than high osmolar contrast media

QUESTION 46

The following statements are true regarding static renal scintigraphy

A. Renal involvemnt during a urinary tract infection can be demonstrated
B. Should not be performed to demonstrate scarring for at least one month following a UTI
C. Images acquired before and after a captopril challenge can be used to demonstrate intrarenal arterial abnormalities
D. Cannot differentiate between deteriorating function in one kidney and increased growth in the other
E. Is not indicated in a child with urinary incontinence

QUESTION 47

Regarding carotid doppler examinations

A. The left vertebral artery originates directly from the aortic arch in 20%
B. Diastolic flow reversal is seen in the common carotid artery
C. Spectral broadening at the carotid bulb is normal
D. The resistive index of the internal carotid artery is twice that of the external carotid artery
E. At the carotid bifurcation, the internal carotid artery usually lies postero-lateral to the external carotid artery

QUESTION 48

Regarding insertion of a nephrostomy tube

A. A bleeding diathesis is an absolute contraindication
B. The risk of death from haemorrhage is 0.2%
C. Gross haematuria for 1-2 days is abnormal
D. Septic shock occurs in 0.1%
E. Haemorrhage can be treated by increasing the nephrostomy tube size

QUESTION 49

The following are true of CT of the paranasal sinuses

A. The nasal cycle alternates every 20-30 minutes
B. Windows of 2000/250 would be appropriate to demonstrate the bony components
C. The osteomeatal complex is best demonstrated on axial scans
D. The turbinates are best demonstrated on coronal scans
E. The cribriform plate is best demonstrated on axial scans

QUESTION 50

The following needle is appropriate to perform a lymphangiogram

A. A 20 gauge McCarthy needle
B. A 30 gauge Rabinov needle
C. A 20 gauge Rabinov needle
D. A 30 gauge McBerni needle
E. A 30 gauge McCarthy needle

QUESTION 51

The following are true of magnetic resonance imaging of the liver

A. Hepatic parenchyma is of higher signal than the spleen on STIR sequences
B. Following ingestion of magnetic iron oxide particles the bowel returns high signal on both T1 and T2 weighted sequences
C. Hepatic vessels are low signal on both T1 and T2 weighted unenhanced sequences
D. Averaging throughout the respiratory cycle reduces movement artefact
E. Respiratory ordered phase-encoding reduces movement artefact

QUESTION 52

Regarding ultrasonography of the spleen

A. The spleen decreases in size with age
B. Visualisation is improved by deep inspiration
C. Visualisation is improved by lying the patient on his right
D. Supernumerary spleens are seen in 30% at autopsy
E. Ultrasound guided biopsy of the spleen is contraindicated

QUESTION 53

Regarding internal biliary drainage

A. Balloon dilatation of benign strictures is contraindicated
B. Plastic stents occlude less frequently than metallic stents
C. Plastic stents are more prone to migration than metallic stents
D. The transhepatic tract is larger for plastic stents than metallic stents
E. Hilar strictures are best treated endoscopically

QUESTION 54

Barium meal double contrast views

A. Supine RAO - antrum
B. Erect - antrum
C. RAO erect - duodenum
D. Prone - body
E. LAO - Caps

QUESTION 55

Regarding the erect AXR

A. A gridded cassette should be used
B. The patient should be standing erect
C. Should be performed in expiration
D. Gonadal protection should routinely be used
E. The use of a slow screen cassette is appropriate

QUESTION 56

Silk Tubes

A. The end hole is for contrast injection
B. Have a titanium weighted tip
C. The stylet needs to be removed to inject contrast
D. Should only use luer lock syringes
E. The internal lumen is coated with water activated lubricant

QUESTION 57

Meckels Diverticulum Radionuclide scan - Drugs administered during

A. Buscopan - 10mgs IV
B. Glucagon - 1mg IV
C. Maxalon - 10mg IV
D. Pentagastrin IV
E. Cimetidine PO

QUESTION 58

Diagnostic catheters are made of

A. Polyurethane
B. Polyethylene
C. Nylon
D. Teflon
E. Polyester

QUESTION 59

Varicography

A. A superficial vein in the foot is punctured
B. The patient should initially be supine
C. The use of a ruler is required
D. A thigh tourniquet is required
E. The patient should ultimately be palced head down

QUESTION 60

TMJ Arthrography

A. 0.3 - 0.6 mls contrast are required
B. Puncture the superior joint space first
C. The head should be flexed laterally
D. Puncture 1 cm behind mandibular condyle
E. Videofluoroscopy may be used

Exam 1: Answers

ANSWER 1
A. TRUE   B. FALSE   C. TRUE   D. TRUE   E. FALSE

The concentration of radioactivity is measured in Bq/ml. Bq/Kg is a measure of the specific activity of a radioactive sample

Gamma rays have a greater maximum possible energy than x-rays. This is because gamma rays originate at a nuclear level whilst x-rays originate from changes in the electron shells

Ref: Curry & Thomas. Christensen's Physics of Diagnostic Radiology. 4th Edition. Williams & Wilkins (Europe) Ltd.

ANSWER 2
A. FALSE   B. TRUE   C. TRUE   D. FALSE   E. TRUE

As the mean kV of the beam is increased with filtration, tissue contrast is reduced

No backing filter is required as the characteristic radiation emitted by the aluminium is of low energy (1.5 kV) and this is absorbed in air

Ref: Curry & Thomas. Christensen's Physics of Diagnostic Radiology. 4th Edition. Williams and Wilkins (Europe) Ltd.

ANSWER 3
A. TRUE   B. TRUE   C. FALSE   D. FALSE   E. TRUE

Z of air is 7.62 and that of the wall is 6. However as the central electrode has a Z of about 13, the Z of the combined ionization chamber (IC) approximates to that of air

In an exposure meter a capacitor is used in parallel to the voltmeter and the central electrode of the chamber is connected to the capacitor

Above a certain wall thickness, the response of the chamber decreases due to attenuation of the beam by the wall itself

The efficiency of detection increases from about 1% to 5% when using a lead cylinder cathode

Ref: Curry & Thomas. Christensen's Physics of Diagnostic Radiology. 4th Edition. Williams and Wilkins (Europe) Ltd.

ANSWER 4
A. FALSE   B. TRUE   C. FALSE   D. TRUE   E. TRUE

The supercoat is usually made of gelatin

The image would be destroyed if the film was exposed to light prior to fixing

Ref: Curry & Thomas. Christensen's Physics of Diagnostic Radiology. 4th Edition. Williams and Wilkins (Europe) Ltd.

ANSWER 5

A. FALSE   B. FALSE   C. FALSE   D. TRUE   E. FALSE

Whilst the use of the oil does provide a degree of filtration and allows the transfer of heat by radiation from the anode, the principal reason that the x-ray tube assembly is immersed in oil is for the electrical insulation it provides.

Ref: Curry & Thomas. Christensen's Physics of Diagnostic Radiology. 4th Edition. Williams & Wilkins (Europe) Ltd.

ANSWER 6

A. TRUE   B. FALSE   C. TRUE   D. FALSE   E. TRUE

The RBE for x-rays is 1

The annual whole body dose limit for a radiation worker is 50 mSv, that for a member of the public is 5 mSv

The average annual whole body dose per person in the UK due to natural background radiation is approximately 2.5 mSv

Ref: Curry & Thomas. Christensen's Physics of Diagnostic Radiology. 4th Edition. Williams & Wilkins (Europe) Ltd.

ANSWER 7

A. FALSE   B. TRUE   C. FALSE   D. TRUE   E. FALSE

The gamma of a film refers to the maximum slope of the straight line portion of the characteristic curve. The steeper the straightline portion the higher the gamma and vice versa

Low gamma film have a wide exposure latitude

The characteristic curve is formed by plotting the optical density against the log of the exposure given to the film

Ref: Armstrong. Lecture Notes on the Physics of Radiology. 1st Edition. 1990. Clinical Press Ltd.

ANSWER 8

A. FALSE   B. TRUE   C. FALSE   D. TRUE   E. TRUE

Immediately following the developer, the film goes straight into the fixer tank after which it is washed with water to remove the silver bromide in solution and fixer chemicals. Fixer has an acid pH of 4-5

Glutaraldehyde is a hardening agent

Ref: Armstrong. Lecture Notes on the Physics of Radiology. 1st Edition. 1990. Clinical Press Ltd.

ANSWER 9

A. TRUE   B. FALSE   C. FALSE   D. FALSE   E. TRUE

Electrons at the periphery of the intensification field are less accurately focused than those at the centre of the magnification field.

This has the following consequences :- the centre of the image intensifier screen has a brighter image, better resolution and less geometric distortion. These features are worse with large field intensifiers

Ref: Armstrong. Lecture Notes on the Physics of Radiology. 1st Edition. 1990. Clinical Press Ltd.

ANSWER 10

A. TRUE   B. FALSE   C. FALSE   D. TRUE   E. TRUE

The amount of heat produced increases with increasing intensity of the U/S beam

Cavitation refers to the formation of bubbles within tissues exposed to ultrasound. It can be either stable or unstable, and tends to be caused more by continuous ultrasound than by intermittent ultrasound

At ultrasound intensities of less than 100 mW per sq. cm, no significant biological effect has been shown to occur in mammals. With increasing intensity, both heat and cavitation are more likely to occur. Cavitation is more likely with high intensity sound at low frequency - unlike the type used in medical ultrasound

Ref: Armstrong. Lecture Notes on the Physics of Radiology. 1st Edition. 1990. Clinical Press Ltd.

ANSWER 11

A. TRUE   B. TRUE   C. FALSE   D. FALSE   E. TRUE

At lower energies, the photoelectric effect is predominant. Hence the interactions are approximately inversely proportional to the cube of the energy

There is no bias toward forward scattering. Scattering can occur in any direction, but in general the larger the angle of deflection of a scattered photon the greater the energy lost by that photon

Ref: Curry & Thomas. Christensen's Physics of Diagnostic Radiology. 4th Edition. Williams & Wilkins (Europe) Ltd.

ANSWER 12

A. FALSE   B. FALSE   C. FALSE   D. FALSE   E. FALSE

Dental x-ray tubes usually use stationary anodes

Fine and coarse focus are selected by energising two different filaments

The greater the angle of swing of an x-ray tube, the thinner the tomographic cut

In multiple simultaneous tomography the film screen combination are of increasing sensitivity

The insulating oil in a rotating anode tube plays an important role in the heat pathway of the rotating anode tubes

Ref: Curry & Thomas. Christensen's Physics of Diagnostic Radiology. 4th Edition. Williams & Wilkins (Europe) Ltd.

ANSWER 13

A. TRUE   B. FALSE   C. FALSE   D. TRUE   E. TRUE

There is a slight bias towards hydrogen nuclei in a spin-up position

A signal can only be detected AFTER a radio frequency pulse is applied

Ref: Curry & Thomas. Christensen's Physics of Diagnostic Radiology. 4th Edition. Williams & Wilkins (Europe) Ltd.

ANSWER 14

A. TRUE   B. TRUE   C. FALSE   D. FALSE   E. FALSE

The use of a grid decreases the amount of scatter reaching the film

The air-gap technique achieves its effect by virtue of scattered photons simply missing the film

At lower kV there tends to be more side scatter production and less scatter in a forward direction

Ref: Farr & Allisy-Roberts. Physics for Medical Imaging. 1st Edition. W B Saunders Co Ltd.

ANSWER 15

A. TRUE   B. TRUE   C. TRUE   D. TRUE   E. TRUE

Ref: Farr & Allisy-Roberts. Physics for Medical Imaging. 1st Edition. W B Saunders Co Ltd.

ANSWER 16

A. FALSE   B. FALSE   C. TRUE   D. FALSE   E. TRUE

A filter is relatively transparent to its own characteristic radiation. The filter serves to remove most of the continuous spectrum.

A single rear screen is used

Compression is vital in order to immobilise the breast, and also to decrease the object to film distance thus decreasing geometric unsharpness

Ref: Farr & Allisy-Roberts. Physics for Medical Imaging. 1st Edition. W B Saunders Co Ltd.

ANSWER 17

A. TRUE   B. FALSE   C. TRUE   D. TRUE   E. FALSE

Annual dose limit for members of the public = 5 mSv

Exceeding 30% of any annual dose limit results in the individual being "classified"

Ref: Farr & Allisy-Roberts. Physics for Medical Imaging. 1st Edition. W B Saunders Co Ltd.

ANSWER 18

A. TRUE   B. FALSE   C. TRUE   D. TRUE   E. FALSE

Near gain: this is poorly named, since it is used primarily to diminish and not enhance near echoes

Reject control discriminates against echoes below a minimum amplitude

Ref: Farr & Allisy-Roberts. Physics for Medical Imaging. 1st Edition. W B Saunders Co Ltd.

ANSWER 19

A. TRUE   B. FALSE   C. TRUE   D. TRUE   E. TRUE

Slice thickness is decreased by increasing the Z field gradient

Ref: Farr & Allisy-Roberts. Physics for Medical Imaging. 1st Edition. W B Saunders Co Ltd.

ANSWER 20

A. FALSE   B. TRUE   C. TRUE   D. FALSE   E. TRUE

GRE: TR-500, TE25, flip angle 40 degrees, would give a T2 weighted image

One of the advantages of gradient echo sequences is that it can be used for volume acquisition of data

Ref: Curry & Thomas. Christensen's Physics of Diagnostic Radiology. 4th Edition. Williams & Wilkins (Europe) Ltd.

ANSWER 21

A. FALSE   B. TRUE   C. FALSE   D. FALSE   E. TRUE

The symphysis menti fuse by 2 years of age

The first permanent molar erupts at six years

Both the upper and lower synovial spaces are not seen in a normal T.M joint arthrogram. This would confirm a disc rupture.

Refs:
Anatomy for Diagnostic Imaging. Ryan & McNicholas. W B Saunders Co Ltd.
Essential Anatomy by Lumley, Craven & Aitken. 3rd Edition. Churchill Livingstone.
Clinical Anatomy by Harold Ellis. 8th Edition. Churchill Livingstone.

ANSWER 22

A. TRUE   B. FALSE   C. FALSE   D. TRUE   E. TRUE

The long saphenous vein enters the femoral vein distal to the inguinal ligament

Although there are more valves below the knee, the long saphenous vein contains several valves in the thigh

Ref:
Last's Anatomy. McMinn. 9th Edition. Churchill Livingstone.

ANSWER 23

A. TRUE   B. FALSE   C. TRUE   D. FALSE   E. TRUE

Popliteus tendon is lateral to the popliteal artery

The posterior tibial artery can be palpated posterior to the medial malleolus

Refs:
Last's Anatomy. McMinn. 9th Edition. Churchill Livingstone.
Anatomy for diagnostic Imaging. Ryan & McNicholas. W B Saunders Co Ltd.

ANSWER 24

A. FALSE   B. FALSE   C. TRUE   D. FALSE   E. TRUE

The joint capsule is attached around the anatomical neck of the humerus

The subacromial bursa does not normally communicate with the shoulder joint

The lateral part of the epiphysis is outside the capsule

Refs:
Last's Anatomy. McMinn. 9th Edition. Churchill Livingstone.
Gray's Anatomy. 38th Edition. Churchill Livingstone.

ANSWER 25

A. TRUE   B. FALSE   C. TRUE   D. FALSE   E. TRUE

The average carpal angle is 135-140 degrees

A sesamoid bone is seen at the thumb interphalangeal joint in approx. 73% of cases

Refs:
Last's Anatomy. McMinn. 9th Edition. Churchill Livingstone.
Anatomy for Diagnostic Imaging. Ryan & McNicholas. W B Saunders Co Ltd.
Atlas of Normal Roentgen Variants. Keats. 6th Edition. Mosby.
An Atlas of Anatomy Basic to Radiology. Meschan. W B Saunders Co Ltd.

ANSWER 26

A. FALSE   B. TRUE   C. FALSE   D. TRUE   E. TRUE

The internal pudendal artery leaves the pelvis via the greater sciatic foramen

The superior rectal artery is a branch of the inferior mesenteric artery

Refs:
Last's Anatomy. McMinn. 9th Edition. Churchill Livingstone.
Gray's Anatomy. 38th Edition. Churchill Livingstone.

ANSWER 27

A. FALSE   B. TRUE   C. TRUE   D. FALSE   E. TRUE

It measures approx. 10 cms in length

The anterior fornix is shallow, the posterior fornix is deep

Refs:
Last's Anatomy. McMinn. 9th Edition. Churchill Livingstone.
Anatomy for Diagnostic Imaging. Ryan & McNicholas. W B Saunders Co Ltd.

ANSWER 28

A. FALSE   B. TRUE   C. FALSE   D. TRUE   E. FALSE

The coeliac artery is the artery of the foregut

The right gastric artery is a branch from the common hepatic artery

The coeliac artery supplies the duodenum up to the mid second part

ANSWER 29

A. TRUE   B. TRUE   C. TRUE   D. TRUE   E. TRUE

Refs:
Last's Anatomy. McMinn. 9th Edition. Churchill Livingstone.
Gray's Anatomy. 38th Edition. Churchill Livingstone.
Anatomy for Diagnostic Imaging. Ryan & McNicholas. W B Saunders Co Ltd.

ANSWER 30

A. FALSE   B. TRUE   C. FALSE   D. FALSE   E. TRUE

Kidneys normally measure between 11-15 cm in length

Pelvic kidneys take blood supply from the internal iliac artery

The renal pelvis is the most posterior structure at the hilum

Refs:
Last's Anatomy. McMinn. 9th Edition. Churchill Livingstone.
Gray's Anatomy. 38th Edition. Churchill Livingstone.

ANSWER 31

A. FALSE   B. FALSE   C. TRUE   D. TRUE   E. FALSE

Lymphoid follicles in the rectum normally measure up to 4 mm in diameter

The post rectal space may measure up to 1.5 cm in length at S4

The portal vein lies anterior to the epiploic foramen

Refs:
Last's Anatomy. McMinn. 9th Edition. Churchill Livingstone.
Gray's Anatomy. 38th Edition. Churchill Livingstone.
An Atlas of Anatomy Basic to Radiology . Meschan. W B Saunders Co Ltd.

ANSWER 32

A. TRUE   B. TRUE   C. FALSE   D. FALSE   E. TRUE

Ligamentum nuchae is represented above level C7.

The ligamentum flavum passes from anterior surface of one lamina to the posterior surface of the lamina below.

Refs:
Anatomy for Diagnostic Imaging. Ryan & McNicholas. W B Saunders Co Ltd.
Essential Anatomy by Lumley, Craven & Aitken. 3rd Edition. Churchill Livingstone.
Clinical Anatomy by Harold Ellis. 8th Edition. Churchill Livingstone.

ANSWER 33

A. FALSE   B. TRUE   C. FALSE   D. TRUE   E. FALSE

The left main bronchus is 5cm long.

The posterior relations of the left main bronchus are oesophagus and descending aorta.

The lingula lobe bronchus comes off the upper lobe bronchus.

Refs:
Anatomy for Diagnostic Imaging. Ryan & McNicholas. W B Saunders Co Ltd.
Essential Anatomy by Lumley, Craven & Aitken. 3rd Edition. Churchill Livingstone.
Clinical Anatomy by Harold Ellis. 8th Edition. Churchill Livingstone.

ANSWER 34

A. TRUE   B. FALSE   C. FALSE   D. FALSE   E. TRUE

The scalenus anterior muscle divides the subclavian artery into 3 parts.

The first part of subclavian artery lies above the lung apex.

The scalenus anterior muscle separates the subclavian artery and vein.

Refs:
Anatomy for Diagnostic Imaging. Ryan & McNicholas. W B Saunders Co Ltd.
Essential Anatomy by Lumley, Craven & Aitken. 3rd Edition. Churchill Livingstone.
Clinical Anatomy by Harold Ellis. 8th Edition. Churchill Livingstone.

ANSWER 35

A. TRUE   B. TRUE   C. FALSE   D. TRUE   E. FALSE

There are 20 deciduous teeth.

The parotid duct pierces the buccinator.

Refs:
Anatomy for Diagnostic Imaging. Ryan & McNicholas. W B Saunders Co Ltd.
Essential Anatomy by Lumley, Craven & Aitken. 3rd Edition. Churchill Livingstone.
Clinical Anatomy by Harold Ellis. 8th Edition. Churchill Livingstone.

ANSWER 36

A. FALSE   B. FALSE   C. TRUE   D. FALSE   E. FALSE

Fourth ventricle is the cavity of hind brain only

The cavity is diamond shaped. The inferior medullary velum lies between the inferior cerebellar peduncles

There is only one median and two lateral openings

Refs:
Anatomy for Diagnostic Imaging. Ryan & McNicholas. W B Saunders Co Ltd.
Essential Anatomy by Lumley, Craven & Aitken. 3rd Edition. Churchill Livingstone.
Clinical Anatomy by Harold Ellis. 8th Edition. Churchill Livingstone.

ANSWER 37
A. TRUE   B. TRUE   C. TRUE   D. FALSE   E. FALSE

The superior and middle thyroid veins and not the inferior thyroid vein drain into the internal jugular vein.

Refs:
Anatomy for Diagnostic Imaging. Ryan & McNicholas. W B Saunders Co Ltd.
Essential Anatomy by Lumley, Craven & Aitken. 3rd Edition. Churchill Livingstone.
Clinical Anatomy by Harold Ellis. 8th Edition. Churchill Livingstone.

ANSWER 38
A. TRUE   B. FALSE   C. TRUE   D. TRUE   E. TRUE

The posterior fontanelle closes by 2-3 months

Refs:
Anatomy for Diagnostic Imaging. Ryan & McNicholas. W B Saunders Co Ltd.
Essential Anatomy by Lumley, Craven & Aitken. 3rd Edition. Churchill Livingstone.
Clinical Anatomy by Harold Ellis. 8th Edition. Churchill Livingstone.

ANSWER 39
A. TRUE   B. TRUE   C. TRUE   D. TRUE   E. TRUE

Refs:
Anatomy for Diagnostic Imaging. Ryan & McNicholas. W B Saunders Co Ltd.
Essential Anatomy by Lumley, Craven & Aitken. 3rd Edition. Churchill Livingstone.
Clinical Anatomy by Harold Ellis. 8th Edition. Churchill Livingstone.

ANSWER 40
A. TRUE   B. TRUE   C. TRUE   D. TRUE   E. TRUE

Refs:
Anatomy for Diagnostic Imaging. Ryan & McNicholas. W B Saunders Co Ltd.
Essential Anatomy by Lumley, Craven & Aitken. 3rd Edition. Churchill Livingstone.
Clinical Anatomy by Harold Ellis. 8th Edition. Churchill Livingstone.

ANSWER 41
A. FALSE   B. FALSE   C. FALSE   D. TRUE   E. TRUE

Compression allows the use of a lower kVp. 26-30 kVp gives the highest soft tissue contrast for a non-grid film-screen system and a Molybdenum target. Higher values required if a grid is used. Single emulsion film is used for all mammography.

Ref: Grainger & Allison. Diagnostic Radiology. 3rd Edition. Churchill Livingstone.

ANSWER 42
A. TRUE   B. TRUE   C. TRUE   D. FALSE   E. FALSE

99mTc-MIBI is trapped by both normal thyroid and normal parathyroid tissue but washes out of thyroid tissue more quickly.

ANSWER 43
A. TRUE   B. TRUE   C. TRUE   D. FALSE   E. FALSE

An occlusal film demonstrates the submandibular ducts. When imaging the parotid with a PA film the head is turned 5 degrees away from the side being studied

Ref: Chapman & Nakielny. A Guide to Radiological Procedures. 3rd Edition. W B Saunders Co Ltd.

ANSWER 44
A. TRUE   B. TRUE   C. TRUE   D. FALSE   E. FALSE

Renal agenesis is more common on the left. Bladder volume is calculated using a factor of 0.7.

Ref: Grainger & Allison. Diagnostic Radiology. 3rd Edition. Churchill Livingstone.

ANSWER 45
A. FALSE   B. TRUE   C. TRUE   D. FALSE   E. TRUE

Calyceal detail is much greater on an IVP than with ultrasound. Low osmolar contrast media delivers a smaller osmotic load so that diuresis is less. Compression therefore is more important with non-ionic contrast media.

Ref: Whitehouse & Worthington. Techniques in Diagnostic Imaging. 3rd Edition. Blackwell Science Ltd.

ANSWER 46
A. TRUE   B. FALSE   C. TRUE   D. FALSE   E. FALSE

A DMSA should be avoided for three months following a UTI to avoid FALSE positives. A DMSA can differentiate between deteriorating function in one kidney and increased growth in the other as it gives an estimate of the mass of functioning cortex. A DMSA is indicated to look for a duplex kidney with ectopic insertion.

Ref: Grainger & Allison. Diagnostic Radiology. 3rd Edition. Churchill Livingstone.

ANSWER 47
A. FALSE   B. FALSE   C. TRUE   D. FALSE   E. TRUE

The left vertebral artery originates from the aortic arch 5%. Continuous forward flow is seen in the common carotid artery. The resistive index of the external carotid artery tends to 1.0 whilst the internal carotid artery tends to 0.5.

Ref: Grainger & Allison. Diagnostic Radiology. 3rd Edition. Churchill Livingstone.

ANSWER 48
A. TRUE   B. TRUE   C. FALSE   D. TRUE   E. TRUE

Gross haematuria can be normal upto 2 days after a nephrostomy insertion.

Ref: Grainger & Allison. Diagnostic Radiology. 3rd Edition. Churchill Livingstone.

ANSWER 49

A. FALSE B. TRUE C. FALSE D. TRUE E. FALSE

Physiological mucosal swelling opens and closes alternate nasal airways every 2-3 hours. Both the osteomeatal complex and the cribriform plate are best demonstrated in the coronal plane.

Ref: Grainger & Allison. Diagnostic Radiology. 3rd Edition. Churchill Livingstone.

ANSWER 50

A. FALSE B. FALSE C. FALSE D. FALSE E. TRUE

20 guage is too large. A 30 guage Rabinov needle is used for sialography.

Ref: Chapman & Nakielny. A Guide to Radiological Procedures. 3rd Edition. W B Saunders Co Ltd.

ANSWER 51

A. FALSE B. FALSE C. TRUE D. TRUE E. TRUE

The spleen returns very high signal on STIR sequences. Magnetic iron oxide particles cause a shortening of both T1 and T2, and bowel appears very low signal on T2W signals.

Ref: Grainger & Allison. Diagnostic Radiology. 3rd Edition. Churchill Livingstone.

ANSWER 52

A. TRUE B. FALSE C. TRUE D. TRUE E. FALSE

Deep inspiration brings the lung down beween the probe and the spleen. Biopsy or drainage is not contraindicated unless there is a bleeding diathesis.

Ref: Grainger & Allison. Diagnostic Radiology. 3rd Edition. Churchill Livingstone.

ANSWER 53

A. FALSE B. FALSE C. TRUE D. TRUE E. FALSE

Plastic stents occlude more frequently because metallic stents are self-expanding and therefore larger in calibre. Percutaneous techniques have a higher success rate for hilar strictures.

Ref: Grainger & Allison. Diagnostic Radiology. 3rd Edition. Churchill Livingstone.

ANSWER 54

A. TRUE B. FALSE C. TRUE D. FALSE E. FALSE

An erect view of the antruum is single contrast. In the prone position contrast obscures the gastric body. The duodenal cap is best demonstrated in the RAO position both supine or semi erect.

Ref: Whitehouse & Worthington. Techniques in Diagnostic Imaging. 3rd Edition. Blackwell Science Ltd.

ANSWER 55

A. TRUE   B. FALSE   C. FALSE   D. FALSE   E. FALSE

The patient can be sitting down. Preferably performed in inspiration. Only men require gonadal protection. A detail or fast screen combination is used.

Ref: Whitehouse & Worthington. Techniques in Diagnostic Imaging. 3rd Edition. Blackwell Science Ltd.

ANSWER 56

A. FALSE   B. FALSE   C. FALSE   D. FALSE   E. TRUE

Silk tubes have no end hole. The tip is made of Tungsten. The fact that contrast can be injected without removing the stylet is one of the advantages of the silk tube. Silk tubes can also accept a bladder syringe with its connection.

Ref: Whitehouse and Worthington. Techniques in Diagnostic Imaging. 3rd Edition. Blackwell Science Ltd.

ANSWER 57

A. FALSE   B. TRUE   C. FALSE   D. FALSE   E. TRUE

Pentagastrin is administered subcutaneously.

Ref. : Chapman & Nakielny. A Guide to Radiological Procedures. 3rd Edition. W B Saunders Co Ltd.

ANSWER 58

A. TRUE   B. TRUE   C. TRUE   D. TRUE   E. FALSE

Ref: Whitehouse & Worthington. Techniques in Diagnostic Imaging. 3rd Edition. Blackwell Science Ltd.

ANSWER 59

A. FALSE   B. FALSE   C. TRUE   D. FALSE   E. TRUE

The varicose vein is punctured. The patient initially starts erect. A ruler is put on the medial aspect of the leg to measure perforating vessels. No tourniquet is usually necessary. The patients head is then tilted down to fill the proximal varicose veins and to find their final drainage site.

Ref: Chapman & Nakielny. A Guide to Radiological Procedures. 3rd Edition. W B Saunders Co Ltd.

ANSWER 60

A. TRUE   B. FALSE   C. TRUE   D. FALSE   E. TRUE

The inferior joint space is injected. Lateral flexion stops overlap of the two TMJs. The needle is advanced onto the posterio-superior aspect of condyle. Videofluoroscopy allows one to visualise full range of movement.

Ref: Chapman & Nakielny. A Guide to Radiological Procedures. 3rd Edition. W B Saunders Co Ltd.

Exam 2

QUESTION 1

Intensifying screens

A. Increase film speed
B. Improve resolution when compared to film exposed directly to x-rays
C. Have an increased modulation transfer function when used with magnification
D. Increase film contrast
E. When using green emitting phosphors, they are associated with a greater cross-over of light compared with the use of blue emitting phosphors

QUESTION 2

Regarding the photoelectric affect

A. The entire energy of the incident photon is transferred to an orbital electron
B. Following the ejection of an electron, the vacancy is filled by an outer shell electron
C. It is the predominant x-ray interaction in iodinated contrast media
D. It is the predominant x-ray interaction in intensifying screens
E. It is the predominant mechanism by which an aluminium filter removes low energy photons

QUESTION 3

Electromagnetic radiation

A. Includes infra-red light
B. Includes radio-waves
C. Can behave both as a wave and as a particle
D. Includes alpha emission
E. Has energy that is proportional to its wavelength

QUESTION 4

Tube rating

A. Is the maximum value of mA that can be achieved for any given value of kV, exposure time and focal spot size
B. It is the limit of power that can be put into the system
C. Is restricted by the amount of heat that builds up in the system
D. Decreases as the focal spot size increases
E. Is equal to 0.7 x kV x mA x seconds for a three phase generator

QUESTION 5

Ionizing radiation (POPUMET) regulations 1998

A. All persons directing an exposure need to be adequately trained in radiation protection matters
B. POPUMET does not apply to scientific research for in vitro studies
C. The responsibility for an exposure lies with the person clinically directing it
D. The ALARA principle does not apply in POPUMET
E. No exposure should be directed unless its introduction produces a positive net benefit

QUESTION 6

Image quality

A. Under good viewing conditions an optical density difference of 0.04 can be seen on an x-ray film
B. "True" fog occurs when the silver halide grains in a film emulsion are developed following an exposure
C. "True" fog is more likely to occur with the use of slow films
D. Increase in the thickness of a part being irradiated results in an increase in the amount of scatter radiation produced
E. It is acceptable for the beam size to be greater than the film size used

QUESTION 7

Regarding interlocks used in fluoroscopy

A. The fluoroscopy interlock prevents screening if the filament is too hot
B. The preparation interlock prevents a relay from being energised if the exposure factors selected could cause tube overload
C. The exposure interlock prevents the exposure relay from being energised without prior initiation of the preparation circuits
D. The guard timer is set to operate if the exposure time exceeds the set time by more than 10%
E. Fluoroscopy is inhibited if the screening time exceeds 10 minutes

QUESTION 8

Regarding subtraction techniques

A. In photographic subtraction, the mask image is produced by using a single emulsion film with a gamma of -2
B. In photographic subtraction the initial mask is known as positive mask
C. In digital subtraction the image used as a mask is electronically subtracted from a subsequent image
D. In digital subtraction it is essential to achieve almost perfect registration between initial and post-contrast images
E. In a digital system, the electronic signals are fed into a digital to analogue converter from where they can then be manipulated

QUESTION 9

The following window levels and window widths would be appropriate for the associated investigation

A. Abdomen : window level (WL) 60, window width (WW) 400
B. Lung: WL -600, WW 1600
C. Bone: WL 800, WW 2000
D. Posterior Fossa : WL 35, WW 150
E. Brain : WL 35, WW 85

QUESTION 10

Regarding the attenuation of monochromatic radiation

A. Decreases the mean energy of the beam
B. Is the fractional reduction in intensity as it traverses an absorber
C. Is exponential
D. Is contributed to by photon absorption
E. Is contributed to by photon scatter

QUESTION 11

The following are true

A. In an x-ray tube, most of the energy of the filament electrons goes to produce x-rays
B. A photoelectron has the same energy as an incident x-ray photon
C. Characteristic K radiation is produced by electrons with energy greater than that of the K absorption edge
D. The output of an x-ray tube is proportional to the mA on the control panel
E. The output of an x-ray tube is independent of whether the rectification is half-wave or full-wave

QUESTION 12

The following statements are true

A. The proton density of CSF is greater than that of grey matter
B. The proton density of white matter is greater than that of grey matter
C. In spin echo sequences, information regarding proton density can also be obtained
D. A time of repetition (TR) of 4,000 ms would be appropriate in the acquisition of a proton density image
E. A TR of 500 ms would be appropriate for the acquisition of a proton density image

QUESTION 13

Secondary radiation grids

- A. Grid ratio equals the ratio of :-[height of the lead strips : width of the lead strips in the grid]
- B. A typical grid ratio used in most diagnostic radiology is 20:1
- C. High ratio grids are preferable at high kVs and with very large field areas
- D. Contrast improvement factor is defined as the contrast obtained with a grid: contrast obtained without a grid
- E. Bucky factor is defined as exposure necessary with a grid : exposure necessary without a grid

QUESTION 14

The following statements regarding image quality are true

- A. Contrast between adjacent areas of a film is due to the difference in their optical densities
- B. Radiographic contrast is defined as the ratio of : film gamma : subject contrast
- C. Screen unsharpness is greatest when using thinner screens
- D. Screen unsharpness can be reduced by using coarser crystals
- E. A high definition screen may typically have an intensification factor of 100

QUESTION 15

Regarding the image intensifier

- A. Zinc cadmium sulphide (ZnCdS) is usually used as the input phosphor
- B. Caesium iodide (CsI) is usually used as the output phosphor
- C. The input phosphor absorbs about 20% of the x-ray energy converting it into light
- D. Photo-electrons produced in the image intensifier are accelerated by a potential difference of 25-35V between the input and output screens
- E. CsI crystals have a higher packing density than ZnCdS crystals resulting in increased screen efficiency

QUESTION 16

The following UK legislation is appropriate for the individuals described

- A. Staff and members of the public: Ionising Radiation Regulations 1985 (IRR 85)
- B. Patients: IRR (POPUMET) 88
- C. Staff and members of the public: Radioactive Substances Act 1993
- D. Patients: The Medicines (Administration of Radioactive Substances) Regulations 1978: M(ARS)R 78
- E. Approved Codes of Practice and Guidance Notes: these do not play a part in UK legislation

QUESTION 17
Regarding ultrasound (U/S)

A. U/S waves may be produced by a transducer containing polyvinylidine difluorine (PVDF)
B. U/S undergoes reflection, but not refraction, at an interface between two different media
C. U/S refers to sound waves of frequency greater than 10,000 Hz
D. A piezoelectric transducer will convert both electrical energy into sound energy and sound energy into electrical energy
E. The Curie temperature refers to the temperature above which a piezoelectric crystal must be heated to in order to produce U/S

QUESTION 18
Regarding ultrasound (U/S)

A. Liquids transmit sound with a wide range of velocities
B. The backing block in an U/S transducer is made of gelatin
C. The Curie temperature of lead zirconate titanate is 570 degrees centigrade
D. The length of the Fresnel zone can be calculated from the product of: square of the diameter of the transducer and the wavelength of sound emitted
E. The length of the Fresnel zone elongates with increasing transducer frequencies

QUESTION 19
Regarding MRI

A. In multi-slice techniques the longer the time to echo (TE) compared to time for repetition (TR), the more slices can be interleaved before repeating the first slice
B. In multi-echo techniques, following each 90 degree pulse, two or more successive 180 degree pulses produce successive echoes with decreasing TE
C. Fat produces a paradoxically high signal on fast spin echo techniques
D. Fast spin echo is a multi-echo technique, in which the sequences are modified by phase encoding each of the echoes with a different encoding gradient
E. The time needed to acquire an image is the product of: (a) the number of excitations and (b) the number of phase encoding steps, divided by (c) the time for repetition (TR)

QUESTION 20
Regarding Gadolinium used as a contrast agent in MRI

A. Is a diamagnetic substance
B. Has paired outer shell electrons
C. Is rendered non-toxic by chelation to DTPA
D. Shortens T1 and prolongs T2
E. Recommended dose is 1mmol per kg = 2ml per kg

QUESTION 21

Regarding the paranasal sinuses

A. The frontal sinus are usually visible by the age of two years
B. Pneumatisation of sphenoid sinus usually occurs at puberty
C. The maxillary sinuses are first to appear and radiologically visualised a few weeks after birth
D. The osteomeatal complex is where the maxillary, frontal and posterior ethmoid sinuses drain
E. MRI is poor in demonstrating the paranasal sinuses

QUESTION 22

Regarding the accessory bones of the foot

A. Os trigonum is seen just anterior to the talus
B. Os peroneum is seen proximal to the base of the 5th metatarsal adjacent to the cuboid
C. Os peroneum may be multicentric
D. Os tibiale externum may be fused to the cuboid
E. Os vesalianum is seen at the base of the 1st metatarsal

QUESTION 23

Regarding the bones of the foot

A. Medial cuneiform articulates with 1st and 2nd metatarsals
B. The lateral cuneiform is the shortest of the three cuneiforms
C. The spring ligament is attached to the inferior margin of the navicular
D. The sustentaculum tali is a projection on the medial side of the talus
E. Ossification centres are present for all three cuneiforms by 4 years

QUESTION 24

In the axilla

A. Teres major is behind the long head of triceps
B. Teres minor is supplied by a subscapular nerve
C. The axillary nerve supplies nothing in the axilla
D. The lateral group of lymph nodes receive lymph from the axillary tail of the breast
E. The axillary artery is divided into three parts by pectoralis minor

QUESTION 25

The radial artery

A. Arises from the brachial artery at the level of the neck of the radius
B. Gives off the anterior interosseous artery
C. Lies on brachioradialis in the upper forearm
D. Lies medial to the superficial branch of the radial nerve in the forearm
E. Forms the deep palmar arch

QUESTION 26
The bladder

A. Is supplied by the obturator artery in its lower part
B. Is covered by peritoneum superiorly
C. Drains to both internal and external iliac lymph nodes
D. The trigone is the area between the ureteral orifices and the external urethral orifice
E. Is drained by veins following the superior and inferior vesical arteries

QUESTION 27
The following statements are true

A. The majority of the female urethra is embedded in the vaginal wall
B. The ampulla of the uterine tube is a dilatation at its outer end
C. The rectouterine pouch is the lowest part of the pelvic peritoneum
D. The infundibulum of the uterine tube is the portion just distal to the uterine opening
E. The uterine tube is supplied by a branch of the ovarian artery

QUESTION 28
Regarding the stomach

A. The gastrooesophageal junction usually lies at the level of T10
B. The incisura angularis is seen on the lesser curve
C. It may be supplied by a branch of the superior mesenteric artery
D. Lymph drainage is partially to nodes at the splenic hilum
E. The gastroduodenal vein drains the greater curvature

QUESTION 29
Concerning the suprarenal glands

A. The right suprarenal gland has a peritoneal covering on its lower half
B. The middle suprarenal artery is multiple in about 5% of cases
C. The right suprarenal gland is higher than the left
D. In cross section, the right suprarenal gland is usually V shaped
E. The left suprarenal gland is related to the medial border of the left kidney

QUESTION 30
The rectus abdominis muscle

A. Is attached to the posterior surface of the pubic bone
B. Is adherent to the posterior rectus sheath at tendinous intersections
C. Is attached to the lower margin of the 6th, 7th and 8th costal cartilages
D. Is related to the superior epigastric artery on its posterior surface
E. Arises by two heads, medial and lateral

QUESTION 31

Regarding the renal tract

A. In a duplex system the upper moiety ureter inserts into the bladder below that draining the lower moiety
B. The indentations of fetal lobation are situated between calyces
C. The left renal vein is retroaortic in 1%
D. The left renal vein splits to surround the aorta in 7%
E. Perinephric fat is most abundant at the upper poles

QUESTION 32

The following statements are true

A. Chamberlain's line joins the posterior tip of the hard palate to the anterior lip of foramen magnum
B. McGregor's line is from the posterior tip of the hard palate to the base of occiput
C. Each typical vertebra has 3 primary and 3 secondary centres of ossification
D. Axis (C2 vertebra) has 2 extra ossification centres when compared to atlas (C1 vertebra)
E. In axial CT intervertebral foramen appear narrower in cuts through its upper and lower ends

QUESTION 33

The following statements are true

A. The oblique fissures extend from T6 posteriorly to the diaphragm anteroinferiorly
B. The left oblique fissure is more vertical in orientation when compared to right
C. The horizontal fissure on the right side is at the level of 4th costal cartilage
D. The horizontal fissure is absent in 30% of normal subjects
E. The azygous fissure has 4 pleural layers and present in 1% of normal individuals

QUESTION 34

The following statements are true

A. The brachiocephalic veins are formed at the mid clavicular region
B. The right brachiocephalic vein lies anterolateral to its artery
C. The left brachiocephalic vein is longer than the right one
D. The superior vena cava is formed behind the junction of the first right costal cartilage with the manubrium
E. The only tributary of superior vena cava is the azygous vein.

QUESTION 35

The following are true

A. The parapharyngeal spaces are filled with air
B. The parapharyngeal spaces are triangular in shape
C. The parapharyngeal spaces are always symmetrical
D. The atlas bone has no foramen transversarium
E. The interspinous distance in the cervical region is maximum between C6 and C7

QUESTION 36

The following are true regarding the spinal cord

A. The spinal cord is about 45cm long
B. The enlargements in the spinal cord lie opposite the lower cervical and lower thoracic vertebrae
C. The collection of all lumbar, sacral and coccygeal nerves is called the filum terminale
D. The posterior median sulcus is deeper than the anterior median fissure
E. The spinal cord is slightly flattened anteroposteriorly

QUESTION 37

Regarding the external ear

A. The auricle is composed of both hyaline and fibrocartilage
B. The external acoustic canal is composed of cartilage in its lateral two thirds and bone in its medial one third
C. The bony part of external auditory meatus is entirely formed by temporal bone
D. The tympanic membrane lies obliquely with its lateral surface facing downwards and forwards
E. The handle of the malleus is attached to the medial surface of tympanic membrane

QUESTION 38

Regarding the mandible

A. The coronoid process gives attachment to medial pterygoid
B. The mandibular foramen lies at the centre of the medial surface of the ramus
C. The sphenomandibular ligament is attached to the lingula
D. The sublingual and submandibular glands are separated by the mylohyoid muscle
E. The digastric fossa lies below the mid-point of the two mylohyoid lines

QUESTION 39

Regarding the limbic lobe

A. It includes the cingulate gyrus, splenial gyrus and dentate gyrus
B. The hippocampus lies in the floor of the inferior horn of the lateral ventricle
C. The posterior end of hippocampus has the appearances of a "paw", also called the peshippocampi
D. The efferent pathway from the hippocampus to the mamillary bodies is called fornix
E. The posterior pillar of the fornix is called the crus of fornix

QUESTION 40

The annulus fibrosus of a intervertebral disc

A. Contains elastic tissue
B. Consists of fibrous layers perpendicular to each other
C. It is attached to the lower vertebra body only
D. Attaches to both anterior and posterior longitudinal ligaments
E. It has no sensory nerve supply

QUESTION 41

Regarding breast ultrasound

A. A 7-10 MHz linear array probe is appropriate
B. Fatty tissue is highly reflective
C. During lactation lactiferous ducts can measure 8 mm in diameter
D. Is useful to evaluate the retro-areolar area
E. Stand-off techniques are required to visualise the skin

QUESTION 42

When imaging the thyroid gland

A. With ^{99m}Tc-pertechnetate, imaging should commence one hour following injection
B. With ^{123}I-sodium iodide imaging should commence at one hour following injection
C. Amiodorone treatment is likely to result in poor uptake
D. The thyroid gland should take up ^{99m}Tc-pertechnetate in a similar way to the salivary glands
E. Potassium perchlorate should be given prior to the study to block the salivary glands

QUESTION 43

Regarding dacrocystography

A. 0.5 to 2.0 mls of contrast is injected each side
B. The superior cannaliculus is preferable
C. A 16 gauge cannula is appropriate
D. Lipiodol is an acceptable contrast media
E. Simultaneous bilateral injections are usually performed

QUESTION 44

Regarding ultrasound of the prostate

A. The transitional zone is hyperechoic
B. The central zone is hyperechoic
C. The peripheral zone is more reflective than the transitional zone
D. The normal prostate is approximately 2.5 cms in AP diameter
E. Seminal vesicles are normally up to 1 cm in width

QUESTION 45

When imaging the renal tract

A. A cross-kidneys film is centred on the ziphisternum and performed in arrested inspiration
B. A 45 degree posterior oblique projection demonstrates the kidneys best
C. Renal tomography is performed at the level of one-third of the AP width of the patient
D. The narrower the angular swing during tomography, the narrower the section
E. The angular swing for nephrotomograms is between 15 and 25 degrees

QUESTION 46

On an occipito-frontal x-ray with 20 degrees of caudal angulation the following can be seen

A. The petrous ridge, seen projected within the orbits
B. The coronal suture
C. The foramen rotundum
D. The foramen ovale
E. The zygomatic arch

QUESTION 47

The umbilical vein

A. Carries oxygenated blood to the inferior vena cava via the ductus venosus
B. Forms the ligamentum teres in the new born
C. Forms the left main portal vein in the new born
D. Forms the ligamentus venosum in the new born
E. Forms the median umbilical ligament

QUESTION 48

Regarding Gallium citrate scans

A. Gallium accumulates in both tumours and infection
B. Localisation of abnormal uptake may require subtraction studies
C. Images are acquired at 6 and 24 hours
D. Gallium is excreted via the liver
E. Is taken up by normal breast tissue

QUESTION 49

Regarding oral cholecystography

A. Gallbladder opacification with iopanoic acid is unaffected by fat malabsorbtion
B. An intravenous cholangiogram within the past week is a contraindication
C. Is contraindicated in acute cholecystitis
D. Is unlikely to be helpful if the serum bilirubin is less 34 micromols/litre
E. Previous cholecystectomy is a contraindication

QUESTION 50

The following are true of computed tomography of the liver

A. The liver is usually around 10 HU less than the spleen in attenuation on unenhanced scans
B. Hepatic parenchyma attenuation peaks at 40-60 seconds after commencing an intravenous injection of contrast
C. The average increase in attenuation of hepatic parenchyma following intravenous contrast media is approximately 80 HU
D. The hepatic vessels are of low attenuation than the parenchyma on unenhanced scans
E. Normally functioning hepatocyte return to their nonenhanced attenuation values by 6 hours following intravenous contrast media

QUESTION 51
When placing an intrahepatic portosystemic shunt

A. The transfemoral approach is used
B. A stent is placed between the portal vein and the IVC
C. Follow up is by ultrasound with doppler
D. Normal portal flow is hepatopedal
E. Normal portal venous flow velocity is 15-18 cm per second

QUESTION 52
Regarding MRI of the liver

A. Magnetic iron oxide particles are taken up predominantly by hepatocytes
B. Following injection of magnetic iron oxide particles normal liver parenchyma returns reduced signal on T2W images
C. Gd-DTPA is taken up predominantly by kupffer cells
D. Optimal imaging following Gd-BOPTA is at 20-30 seconds following injection
E. Following injection of Gadolinium chelate the timing of liver enhancement parallels that of dynamic CT

QUESTION 53
Endoscopy

A. Upper GI - perforation rate of 0.1%
B. High dysphagia is a contraindication
C. Cricopharyngeal region is well demonstrated
D. Cricropharyngeus is approx 15 cms from incisors
E. Gastroesophageal junction is approximately 25 cms from cricopharyngeus

QUESTION 54
Small bowel enema

A. Incurs a higher radiation dose than a small bowel meal
B. Contraindicated in small bowel obstruction
C. Excellent for detecting perforations
D. Apply local anaesthesia to nostril
E. Apply local anaesthesia to throat

QUESTION 55
Vascular catheters - the following statements are true

A. Polyurethane catheters are stiffer than polyethylene
B. Polyethelene catheters are used with a teflon coated wire
C. Pigtail catheters have end holes
D. Pigtail catheters have side holes in the curved portion
E. Polyethylene catheters are softer than polyurethane

QUESTION 56
Coronary Angiography positions adopted in

A. Left main stem - right lateral
B. Left main stem - RAO
C. Right coronary - AP
D. Right coronary - RAO
E. LAD - AP

QUESTION 57
Radionuclide bone scan

A. Maximum dose of 100 MBq
B. Uses HMPAO
C. Uses MDP
D. Uses ^{99m}Tc
E. Uses pertechnetate

QUESTION 58
The following centering points are correct

A. Oblique hand - 3rd metacarpal head
B. Ball-catchers hand - 5th metacarpal head
C. Lateral wrist - radial styloid
D. PA wrist - midshaft 3rd metacarpal
E. Lateral elbow - 2.5 cms inferior to lateral epicondyle

QUESTION 59
Regarding tenography

A. The needle is inserted under screening
B. MRI has better resolution
C. Contrast is injected to confirm position
D. 5-10 mls of 0.5% Bupivicaine is injected
E. Tenography is predominantly a therapeutic procedure

QUESTION 60
The following are contraindications to bronchography

A. Bleeding diathesis
B. Asthma
C. Acute chest infection
D. Recent bronchoscopy
E. Poor respiratory reserve

Exam 2: Answers

ANSWER 1
A. TRUE   B. FALSE   C. TRUE   D. TRUE   E. TRUE

The image is affected by screen unsharpness and consequently has a lower resolution compared to film exposed directly

Film contrast is increased because screens diminish the effect of scatter when compared to film exposed alone

Ref: Curry & Thomas. Christensen's Physics of Diagnostic Radiology. 4th Edition. Williams and Wilkins (Europe) Ltd.

ANSWER 2
A. TRUE   B. TRUE   C. TRUE   D. TRUE   E. TRUE

Ref: Curry & Thomas. Christensen's Physics of Diagnostic Radiology. 4th Edition. Williams and Wilkins (Europe) Ltd.

ANSWER 3
A. TRUE   B. TRUE   C. TRUE   D. FALSE   E. FALSE

Alpha emission is particulate emission from radioactive decay

The energy of electromagnetic radiation is inversely proportional to its wave length and derived from the equation $E = hc/\lambda$

Ref: Curry & Thomas. Christensen's Physics of Diagnostic Radiology. 4th Edition. Williams & Wilkins (Europe) Ltd.

ANSWER 4
A. TRUE   B. TRUE   C. TRUE   D. FALSE   E. FALSE

The tube rating tends to increase with increase in focal spot size

Three phase generators are about 35% more efficient than single phase generators. Thus the tube rating for a three phase unit is equal to 1.35 x kV x mA x seconds

Ref: Curry & Thomas. Christensen's Physics of Diagnostic Radiology. 4th Edition. Williams & Wilkins (Europe) Ltd.

ANSWER 5
A. TRUE   B. TRUE   C. TRUE   D. FALSE   E. TRUE

The ALARA principle should always be applied when directing ionizing radiation

Ref: Curry & Thomas. Christensen's Physics of Diagnostic Radiology. 4th Edition. Williams & Wilkins (Europe) Ltd.

ANSWER 6
A. TRUE   B. FALSE   C. FALSE   D. TRUE   E. FALSE

An optical density of 0.04 equates to a difference in light transmission of 10%

"True" fog occurs when the silver halide grains in an emulsion are developed in the absence of exposure to light or x-rays

"True" fog is more likely to be seen with the use of high-speed films due to their highly sensitised grains

It is good radiological practice for the beam size to be less than the film size used, and as such evidence of collimation should be seen on every exposed film

Ref: Armstrong. Lecture Notes on the Physics of radiology. 1st Edition. 1990. Clinical Press Ltd.

ANSWER 7
A. TRUE   B. TRUE   C. TRUE   D. FALSE   E. TRUE

The guard timer terminates an exposure if the exposure time exceeds the set time by 1%

By UK law fluoroscopy is inhibited if screening time exceeds 10 minutes. In practice there is a 5 minute reminder

Ref: Armstrong. Lecture Notes on the Physics of Radiology. 1st Edition. 1990. Clinical Press Ltd.

ANSWER 8
A. FALSE   B. TRUE   C. TRUE   D. TRUE   E. FALSE

The single emulsion used for the mask image has a gamma of -1

It is known as a positive mask because if it is superimposed on the original radiograph all the information is "masked out"

The electronic signals are fed into an analogue to digital converter to produce digital signals which are then manipulated

Ref: Armstrong. Lecture Notes on the Physics of Radiology. 1st Edition. 1990. Clinical Press Ltd.

ANSWER 9
A. TRUE   B. TRUE   C. TRUE   D. TRUE   E. TRUE

These values are used in a CT unit in my department. They are essentially appropriate for the investigations described but the values in your department may differ slightly

ANSWER 10
A. FALSE   B. TRUE   C. TRUE   D. TRUE   E. TRUE

Attenuation of a monochromatic beam by an absorber does not change the quality of the beam but reduces the number of photons in the beam i.e. there is a decrease in quantity of photons

Ref: Curry & Thomas. Christensen's Physics of Diagnostic Radiology. 4th Edition. Williams & Wilkins (Europe) Ltd.

ANSWER 11
A. FALSE   B. FALSE   C. TRUE   D. TRUE   E. FALSE

Only 1% of the energy of electrons goes to produce x-rays. The rest is liberated as heat

A photoelectron has less energy than the incident photon

Tube loading is 35% more efficient with full-wave rectification

Ref: Armstrong. Lecture Notes on the Physics of Radiology. 1st Edition. Clinical Press Ltd.

ANSWER 12
A. TRUE   B. FALSE   C. TRUE   D. TRUE   E. FALSE

Grey matter contains more protons than white matter and thus its proton density is greater

A TR of 500 milliseconds would be appropriate for the acquisition of a T1 weighted image

Ref: Armstrong. Lecture Notes on the Physics of Radiology. 1st Edition. Clinical Press Ltd.

ANSWER 13
A. FALSE   B. FALSE   C. TRUE   D. TRUE   E. FALSE

Grid ratio is a ratio of the height of the lead strips to the distance between them

A typical grid ratio is 8:1

High ratio grids are preferable at high kV's and with very large field areas because more scatter is produced in this setting

The ratio of exposure necessary with a grid to that without a grid describes grid factor. Bucky factor = incident radiation : transmitted radiation

Ref: Farr & Allisy-Roberts. Physics for Medical Imaging. 1st Edition. W B Saunders Co Ltd.

ANSWER 14
A. TRUE   B. FALSE   C. FALSE   D. FALSE   E. FALSE

Radiographic contrast = film gamma x subject contrast

Screen unsharpness is greatest for thicker screens

Screen unsharpness is reduced with screens composed of fine crystals

A high definition screen or "detail" screen typically has an intensification factor of 35

Ref: Farr & Allisy-Roberts. Physics for Medical Imaging. 1st Edition. W B Saunders Co Ltd.

ANSWER 15
A. FALSE   B. FALSE   C. FALSE   D. FALSE   E. TRUE

CsI is usually used as the input phosphor

ZnCdS is usually used as the output phosphor

The input phosphor absorbs about 60% of the x-ray energy

A potential difference of 25-35kV is applied between the input and output Phosphors

CsI has needle-like crystals which can be aligned and packed tightly together

Ref: Farr & Allisy-Roberts. Physics for Medical Imaging. 1st Edition. W B Saunders Co Ltd.

ANSWER 16
A. TRUE   B. TRUE   C. TRUE   D. TRUE   E. FALSE

The approved Codes of Practice and Guidance give detailed and practical recommendations on how the legislation should be implemented locally in x-ray and nuclear medicine departments

Ref: Farr & Allisy-Roberts. Physics for Medical Imaging. 1st Edition. W B Saunders Co Ltd.

ANSWER 17
A. TRUE   B. FALSE   C. FALSE   D. TRUE   E. FALSE

PVDF is a piezoelectric material. Lead zirconate titanate (PZT) is also frequently used

U/S undergoes both reflection and refraction

U/S refers to sound waves of frequency greater than 20 kHz, so as to be inaudible to the human ear

At the Curie temperature, the transducer loses its piezoelectric properties (e.g. 350 degrees centigrade for PZT)

Ref: Farr & Allisy-Roberts. Physics for Medical Imaging. 1st Edition. W B Saunders Co Ltd.

ANSWER 18
A. FALSE   B. FALSE   C. FALSE   D. FALSE   E. TRUE

As the velocity of sound is inversely related to the compressibility of the conducting medium, consequently all liquids transmit sound with a narrow range of velocities

The backing block is made of Tungsten and rubber powders in an epoxy resin

The Curie temperature of PZT = 350 degrees centigrade; Quartz = 570 degrees centigrade

The length of the Fresnel zone (Near zone) = square of the diameter of the transducer divided by the wavelength of sound emitted

Ref: Farr & Allisy-Roberts. Physics for Medical Imaging. 1st Edition. W B Saunders Co Ltd.

ANSWER 19
A. FALSE   B. FALSE   C. TRUE   D. TRUE   E. FALSE

In multi-slice techniques, a succession of 90 and 180 degree radio frequency pulses, each of a different frequency, is delivered in each TR cycle. Thus the shorter the TE is compared to TR, the more the slices can be interleaved in this way

In multi-echo techniques, the echoes are of increasing TE, their peak amplitudes decrease with the time constant T2

The imaging time is found by multiplying the three variables (a), (b) and (c)

Ref: Farr & Allisy-Roberts. Physics for Medical Imaging. 1st Edition. W B Saunders Co Ltd.

ANSWER 20
A. FALSE   B. FALSE   C. TRUE   D. FALSE   E. FALSE

Para-magnetic substance

Has unpaired outer shell electrons

Shortens both T1 and to a lesser extent T2

Recommended dose: 0.1mmol per kg = 0.2ml per kg

Ref: Farr & Allisy-Roberts. Physics for Medical Imaging. 1st Edition. W B Saunders Co Ltd.

ANSWER 21
A. FALSE   B. FALSE   C. TRUE   D. FALSE   E. FALSE

The frontal sinuses are usually not visible until two years

Pneumatisation of sphenoid sinus occurs at the age of three years

Osteomeatal complex is where the maxillary, frontal and anterior ethmoids drain

MRI is surprisingly good at demonstrating the sinuses since the bony septae have no signals outlined by high signal mucosa.

Refs:
Anatomy for Diagnostic Imaging. Ryan & McNicholas. W B Saunders Co Ltd.
Essential Anatomy by Lumley, Craven & Aitken. 3rd Edition. Churchill Livingstone.
Clinical Anatomy by Harold Ellis. 8th Edition. Churchill Livingstone.

ANSWER 22
A. FALSE   B. TRUE   C. TRUE   D. FALSE   E. FALSE

Os trigonum is posterior to the talus

Os tibiale externum may be fused to the navicular

Os vesalianum is seen at the base of the 5th metatarsal

Refs:
Anatomy for Diagnostic Imaging. Ryan & McNicholas. W B Saunders Co Ltd.
Atlas of Normal Roentgen Variants. Keats. 6th Edition. Mosby.

ANSWER 23
A. TRUE   B. FALSE   C. TRUE   D. FALSE   E. TRUE

The Intermediate cuneiform is the shortest of the three cuneiforms

The sustentaculum tali is a projection of the calcaneum

Refs:
Last's Anatomy. McMinn. 9th Edition. Churchill Livingstone.
Anatomy for Diagnostic Imaging. Ryan & McNicholas. W B Saunders Co Ltd.

ANSWER 24
A. FALSE   B. FALSE   C. TRUE   D. FALSE   E. TRUE

Teres major is anterior to the long head of triceps

Teres minor is supplied by a posterior branch of the axillary nerve

The axillary tail drains to posterior axillary nodes

Refs:
Last's Anatomy. McMinn. 9th Edition. Churchill Livingstone.
Gray's Anatomy. 38th Edition. Churchill Livingstone.

ANSWER 25
A. TRUE   B. FALSE   C. FALSE   D. TRUE   E. TRUE

The anterior interosseous artery is a branch of the ulnar artery

Brachioradialis lies over the radial artery in the upper forearm

Refs:
Last's Anatomy. McMinn. 9th Edition. Churchill Livingstone.
Gray's Anatomy. 38th Edition. Churchill Livingstone.

ANSWER 26
A. TRUE   B. TRUE   C. TRUE   D. FALSE   E. FALSE

The trigone is the area between the ureteral orifices and internal urethral orifice

The veins draining the bladder form a plexus around the bladder neck

Refs:
Last's Anatomy. McMinn. 9th Edition. Churchill Livingstone.
Gray's Anatomy. 38th Edition. Churchill Livingstone.

ANSWER 27
A. TRUE   B. TRUE   C. TRUE   D. FALSE   E. TRUE

The infundibulum is at the distal end of the uterine tube

Refs:
Last's Anatomy. McMinn. 9th Edition. Churchill Livingstone.
Anatomy for Diagnostic Imaging. Ryan & McNicholas. W B Saunders Co Ltd.

ANSWER 28
A. TRUE   B. TRUE   C. FALSE   D. TRUE   E. FALSE

The stomach is supplied by branches of the coeliac artery only

There is no gastroduodenal vein

Refs:
Last's Anatomy. McMinn. 9th Edition. Churchill Livingstone.
Gray's Anatomy. 38th Edition. Churchill Livingstone.

ANSWER 29
A. TRUE   B. FALSE   C. FALSE   D. TRUE   E. TRUE

The middle suprarenal artery is multiple in greater than 30% of cases

The left gland normally lies higher than the right

Refs:
Last's Anatomy. McMinn. 8th Edition. Churchill Livingstone.
Gray's Anatomy. 38th Edition. Churchill Livingstone.
Anatomy for Diagnostic Imaging. Ryan & McNicholas. W B Saunders Co Ltd.

ANSWER 30
A. FALSE   B. FALSE   C. FALSE   D. TRUE   E. TRUE

Rectus abdominis is attached to the front of the pubic bone

Rectus abdominis is adherent to the anterior rectus sheath

Rectus abdominis is attached to the 5th, 6th and 7th costal cartilages

Ref:
Last's Anatomy. McMinn. 9th Edition. Churchill Livingstone.
Gray's Anatomy. 38th Edition. Churchill Livingstone.

ANSWER 31
A. TRUE   B. TRUE   C. FALSE   D. TRUE   E. FALSE

The left renal vein is retroaortic in 3.5 %

Perinephric fat is most abundant at the lower poles

Refs:
Last's Anatomy. McMinn. 9th Edition. Churchill Livingstone.
Anatomy for Diagnostic Imaging. Ryan & McNicholas. W B Saunders Co Ltd.

ANSWER 32
A. FALSE   B. TRUE   C. FALSE   D. TRUE   E. TRUE

Chamberlain's line joins the posterior tip of hard palate to the posterior lip of foramen magnum and less than 2mm of the odontoid is normally seen above this.

Each typical vertebra has 3 primary and 5 secondary centres of ossification.

Resf:
Anatomy for Diagnostic Imaging. Ryan & McNicholas, W B Saunders Co Ltd.
Essential Anatomy by Lumley, Craven & Aitken. 3rd Edition. Churchill Livingstone.
Clinical Anatomy by Harold Ellis. 8th Edition. Churchill Livingstone.

ANSWER 33

A. FALSE   B. TRUE   C. TRUE   D. FALSE   E. TRUE

The oblique fissures extend from T4/5 and not T6.

The horizontal fissure is absent in only 10% of subjects.

Refs:
Anatomy for Diagnostic Imaging. Ryan & McNicholas. W B Saunders Co Ltd.
Essential Anatomy by Lumley, Craven & Aitken. 3rd Edition. Churchill Livingstone.
Clinical Anatomy by Harold Ellis. 8th Edition. Churchill Livingstone.

ANSWER 34

A. FALSE   B. TRUE   C. TRUE   D. TRUE   E. TRUE

The brachiocephalic veins are formed at the medial end of the clavicle.

Refs:
Anatomy for Diagnostic Imaging. Ryan & McNicholas. W B Saunders Co Ltd.
Essential Anatomy by Lumley, Craven & Aitken. 3rd Edition. Churchill Livingstone.
Clinical Anatomy by Harold Ellis. 8th Edition. Churchill Livingstone.

ANSWER 35

A. FALSE   B. TRUE   C. FALSE   D. FALSE   E. FALSE

The parapharyngeal spaces are filled with soft tissue contents like lymphoid tissue but not air.

The parapharyngeal spaces can be asymmetrical.

The atlas does have a foramen transversarium.

The maximum interspinous distance is between C2 and C3.

Refs:
Anatomy for Diagnostic Imaging. Ryan & McNicholas. W B Saunders Co Ltd.
Essential Anatomy by Lumley, Craven & Aitken. 3rd Edition. Churchill Livingstone.
Clinical Anatomy by Harold Ellis. 8th Edition. Churchill Livingstone.

ANSWER 36

A. TRUE   B. TRUE   C. FALSE   D. FALSE   E. TRUE

The filum terminale does not include all the lumbar nerves but only the lower lumbar nerves

The anterior median fissure is deeper than posterior median sulcus

Refs:
Anatomy for Diagnostic Imaging. Ryan & McNicholas. W B Saunders Co Ltd.
Essential Anatomy by Lumley, Craven & Aitken. 3rd Edition. Churchill Livingstone.
Clinical Anatomy by Harold Ellis. 8th Edition. Churchill Livingstone.

ANSWER 37

A. FALSE   B. FALSE   C. TRUE   D. TRUE   E. TRUE

The auricle is composed only of fibrocartilage

External acoustic meatus is composed of cartilage in its lateral one third and bone in its medial two thirds

Refs:
Anatomy for Diagnostic Imaging. Ryan & McNicholas. W B Saunders Co Ltd.
Essential Anatomy by Lumley,Craven & Aitken. 3rd Edition. Churchill Livingstone.
Clinical Anatomy by Harold Ellis. 8th Edition. Churchill Livingstone.

ANSWER 38
A. FALSE   B. TRUE   C. TRUE   D. TRUE   E. TRUE

The coronoid process gives attachment to the temporalis muscle

Refs:
Anatomy for Diagnostic Imaging. Ryan & McNicholas. W B Saunders Co Ltd.
Essential Anatomy by Lumley,Craven & Aitken. 3rd Edition. Churchill Livingstone.
Clinical Anatomy by Harold Ellis. 8th Edition. Churchill Livingstone.

ANSWER 39
A. TRUE   B. TRUE   C. FALSE   D. TRUE   E. TRUE

The anterior end of hippocampus forms the peshippocampi

Refs:
Anatomy for Diagnostic Imaging. Ryan & McNicholas. W B Saunders Co Ltd.
Essential Anatomy by Lumley,Craven & Aitken. 3rd Edition. Churchill Livingstone.
Clinical Anatomy by Harold Ellis. 8th Edition. Churchill Livingstone.

ANSWER 40
A. FALSE   B. TRUE   C. FALSE   D. TRUE   E. FALSE

The annulus does not contain elastic tissue

The annulus attaches to both the upper and lower vertebra bodies

It has no motor supply

Refs:
Anatomy for Diagnostic Imaging. Ryan & McNicholas. W B Saunders Co Ltd.
Essential Anatomy by Lumley,Craven & Aitken. 3rd Edition. Churchill Livingstone.
Clinical Anatomy by Harold Ellis. 8th Edition. Churchill Livingstone.

ANSWER 41
A. TRUE   B. FALSE   C. TRUE   D. FALSE   E. TRUE

Fatty tissue is poorly reflective. Acoustic shadows are generated by the dense connective tissue around lactiferous ducts making it difficult to evaluate the retro-areolar area.

Ref: Grainger & Allison. Diagnostic Radiology. 3rd Edition. Churchill Livingstone.

ANSWER 42
A. FALSE   B. FALSE   C. TRUE   D. FALSE   E. FALSE

Imaging starts at 15 minutes following injection of ^{99m}Tc-pertechnetate and 3-4 hours following injection of ^{123}I-sodium iodide. If thyroid uptake is similar to the salivary glands this suggests hypothyroidism. Potassium perchlorate would also cause a thyroid blockade.

Ref: Chapman & Nakielny. A Guide to Radiological Procedures. 3rd Edition. W B Saunders Co Ltd.

ANSWER 43
A. TRUE   B. FALSE   C. FALSE   D. TRUE   E. TRUE

Inferior cannaliculus is preferably cannulated with an 18 gauge cannula.

Ref: Chapman & Nakielny. A Guide to Radiological Procedures. 3rd Edition. W B Saunders Co Ltd.

ANSWER 44
A. FALSE   B. TRUE   C. TRUE   D. TRUE   E. TRUE

The transitional zone is hypoechoic and cannot be separated from the central zone

Ref: Grainger & Allison. Diagnostic Radiology. 3rd Edition. Churchill Livingstone.

ANSWER 45
A. FALSE   B. FALSE   C. TRUE   D. FALSE   E. FALSE

The centering point for a cross-kidneys film is the lower costal margin, and a film is performed in expiration. A 35 degree posterior oblique projection demonstrates the kidneys best. The narrower the angular swing the thicker the section in tomography. The angle of swing is usually between 25-40 degrees.

Ref: Chapman & Nakielny. A Guide to Radiological Procedures. 3rd Edition. W B Saunders Co Ltd.

ANSWER 46
A. FALSE   B. TRUE   C. TRUE   D. FALSE   E. FALSE

The petrous ridge should be level with the lower margin of the orbit, and the beam emerges through the nasion. The petrus ridge is seen within the orbits on an untilted occipito-frontal projection, where the beam emerges through the glabella.

Ref: Bell and Finlay. Basic Radiographic Positioning and Anatomy. 1st Edition. Bailliere Tindall.

ANSWER 47
A. TRUE   B. TRUE   C. TRUE   D. TRUE   E. FALSE

The umbilical arteries form the superior vesical arteries and the medial umbilical ligaments.

Ref: Grainger & Allison. Diagnostic Radiology. 3rd Edition. Churchill Livingstone.

ANSWER 48
A. TRUE   B. TRUE   C. FALSE   D. TRUE   E. TRUE

Subtraction studies of renal scans or liver and spleen colloid scan may be required. Images are aquired at 48 and 72 hours.

Ref: Grainger and Allison. Diagnostic Radiology. 3rd Edition. Churchill Livingstone.

ANSWER 49
A. FALSE   B. TRUE   C. TRUE   D. FALSE   E. TRUE

Iopanoic acid requires fat in the diet for absorbtion. In acute cholecystitis the gall bladder may fail to opacify as E-coli causes deconjugation of the contrast media in the gallbladder, to a form that is rapidly reabsorbed. The serum bilirubin should be less than 34 micromols/litre.

Ref: Chapman & Nakielny. A Guide to Radiological Procedures. 3rd Edition. W B Saunders Co Ltd.

ANSWER 50
A. FALSE   B. TRUE   C. FALSE   D. TRUE   E. FALSE

The liver is 8-10 HU higher than the spleen due to glycogen and iron

The average increase in density of the liver following contrast is around 45 HU, but this does depend on contrast rate volume and osmolality. Normally functioning hepatocytes remain hyperdense at 6 hours following contrast injection, and a delayed scan can be a useful adjunct in the detection of metastases.

Ref: Grainger & Allison. Diagnostic Radiology. 3rd Edition. Churchill Livingstone.

ANSWER 51
A. FALSE   B. FALSE   C. TRUE   D. TRUE   E. TRUE

The transjugular approach is used. The stent is placed between a hepatic vein and an intrahepatic portal vein.

Ref: Grainger & Allison. Diagnostic Radiology. 3rd Edition. Churchill Livingstone.

ANSWER 52
A. FALSE   B. TRUE   C. FALSE   D. FALSE   E. TRUE

Magnetic iron oxide particles are taken up by Kupffer cells. Gd-DTPA is protein bound, and taken up by hepatocytes. Gd-BOPTA is protein bound and taken up by hepatocytes and optimally imaged at 30-60 minutes.

Ref: Grainger & Allison. Diagnostic Radiology. 3rd Edition. Churchill Livingstone.

ANSWER 53
A. FALSE   B. TRUE   C. FALSE   D. TRUE   E. TRUE

The perforation rate of an upper GI endoscopy is 0.018%. Need to exclude a pharyngeal pouch in highdysphagia before performing an endoscopy. The cricopharyngeal region is particularly difficult to visualise by endoscopy.

ANSWER 54
A. TRUE   B. FALSE   C. FALSE   D. TRUE   E. FALSE

Screening time is increased and more spot views are taken during a SB enema than a SB meal. Barium suspension can be used in SB obstruction. Perforation is an absolute contraindication in view of the dangers of barium in the peritoneum. Nasal anaesthesia is helpful for nasal intubations. It is somewhat dangerous to anaesthetise the throat in view of the risk of aspiration if the patient vomits.

Ref: Whitehouse & Worthington. Techniques in Diagnostic Imaging. 3rd Edition. Blackwell Science Ltd.

ANSWER 55
A. TRUE   B. FALSE   C. TRUE   D. FALSE   E. TRUE

Teflon coated wires are used because they have a higher coefficient of friction. The side holes of pigtail catheters are in the straight portion, pigtail catheters with holes on the curved portion are drainage catheters.

Ref: Whitehouse & Worthington. Techniques in Diagnostic Imaging. 3rd Edition. Blackwell Science Ltd.

ANSWER 56
A. FALSE   B. TRUE   C. TRUE   D. TRUE   E. TRUE

The left main stem is demonstrated by a left lateral view.

Ref: Chapman & Nakielny. A Guide to Radiological Procedures. 3rd Edition. W B Saunders Co Ltd.

ANSWER 57
A. FALSE   B. FALSE   C. TRUE   D. TRUE   E. FALSE

The maximum dose is 500-600 MBq.

Ref: Chapman & Nakielny. A Guide to Radiological Procedures. 3rd Edition. W B Saunders Co Ltd.

ANSWER 58
A. FALSE   B. TRUE   C. TRUE   D. FALSE   E. FALSE

An oblique view of the hand is centered on the 5th metacarpal head, PA view of the wrist is centered midway between radial and ulnar styloid, and a lateral view of the elbow is centered on the lateral epicondyle.

Ref: Bell & Finlay. Basic Radiographic Positioning & Anatomy. 1st Edition. Bailliere Tindall.

ANSWER 59

A. FALSE   B. FALSE   C. TRUE   D. TRUE   E. TRUE

The needle is inserted under palpation. Tenography can show very fine irregularity in detail of the tendon not seen on MRI. Free flow of contrast away from the needle tip confirms correct site of puncture. If symptoms resolve with Bupivicaine it confirms the diagnostic problem. MRI and to a lesser extent CT have taken over the diagnosis of tenosynovitis.

Ref: Chapman & Nakielny. A Guide to Radiological Procedures. 3rd Edition. W B Saunders Co Ltd.

ANSWER 60

A. FALSE   B. FALSE   C. TRUE   D. FALSE   E. TRUE

Asthmatics should use steroid prophylaxis and inhalers preoperatively. Bronchoscopy can cause reversible dilatation of the airways which can mimic bronchiectasis.

Ref: Chapman & Nakielny. A Guide to Radiological Procedures. 3rd Edition. W B Saunders Co Ltd.

Exam 3

QUESTION 1

Rare earth screens

A. Allow a lower tube loading
B. Allow the use of smaller focal spots
C. Produce less movement blur
D. Produce less geometric distortion
E. Reduce quantum mottle

QUESTION 2

Regarding the photoelectric effect

A. Both "free" and "bound" electrons are involved
B. Is greater in aluminium than in lead for a given photon energy
C. Results in the emission of characteristic radiation
D. A positron may be emitted
E. Produces significant scatter radiation in the diagnostic energy range

QUESTION 3

Regarding the x-ray tube and x-ray production

A. The focusing cup of the cathode is designed so as to concentrate the electrons on the focal spot
B. A tungsten rhenium target is tougher and less likely to crack due to heating than a target made of tungsten alone
C. A dual focus tube has two filaments of differing sizes which enables the production of two different sizes of focal spot
D. The tube current is measured in volts
E. A rotating anode tube has a significantly higher rating than a tube which has a stationary anode

QUESTION 4

The following are true of Alpha particles

A. They are identical to helium nuclei
B. They travel relatively quickly through matter
C. They produce a relatively small amount of ionization per unit length of track
D. They tend to travel only short distances in solid material
E. They serve no useful purpose in diagnostic radiography

QUESTION 5
Regarding grids and grid cut off

A. Lateral decentering produces a radiograph that is light on one side and dark on the other side
B. Focus grid distance decentering produces a uniformly light radiograph
C. Combined lateral and focus grid distance decentering produces a radiograph that is light at the periphery
D. Combined lateral and focus grid distance decentering is the commonest type of grid of cut off encountered in every day practice
E. Moving grids incur an increased patient radiation dose compared to static grids

QUESTION 6
Regarding tomography

A. Wide angle tomography is also known as zonography
B. The use of wide angle tomography would be effective for imaging the inner ear
C. Narrow angle tomography is useful for imaging tissues with a lot of natural contrast
D. Phantom images tend to be produced more frequently in narrow angle tomography
E. Narrow angle tomography achieves its effects by utilising maximal blurring of obscuring shadows

QUESTION 7
Concerning the isotopes of iodine

A. ^{123}I has a half life of 13 days
B. ^{131}I has a half life of 8 days
C. ^{125}I is a beta emitter
D. A low energy general purpose collimator is used with ^{123}I
E. A high energy general purpose collimator is used with ^{131}I

QUESTION 8
Radiographic contrast depends upon

A. The inherent film contrast
B. Film fog
C. Scatter radiation
D. Subject contrast
E. The conditions under which the film is developed

QUESTION 9

Radiation protection

A. In the UK the average annual total effective dose (ED) to the population is 2.5 Sv
B. 5% of the average annual total ED is from medical investigations or treatment
C. Medical staff in a radiology department commonly receive an annual total ED twice that of the national average
D. Potassium-40 is a major contributor to the ED from background radiaion arising through the ground
E. The residents in Cornwall receive an annual total ED seven times the national average

QUESTION 10

Regarding the linear attenuation coefficient (LAC)

A. Of tissue, is dependent on the density of the tissue
B. For monochromatic radiation the LAC is inversely proportional to the half value layer of the tissue
C. Of an absorber, is greater for a high energy beam than it is for a low energy beam
D. Of fat, is greater than the LAC of muscle within the diagnostic energy range
E. Has units - per meter

QUESTION 11

Regarding the production of x-rays

A. Tungsten may be used as the material in either the cathode or the anode
B. Tungsten is used as the target material primarily due to its high thermal conductivity
C. The mA is controlled by varying the filament temperature
D. The quality of an x-ray beam depends upon the square of the kVp, mAs, atomic number and wave form
E. X-ray production is 99% efficient

QUESTION 12

The following statements are true

A. Total unsharpness = square root of [geometric unsharpness squared + movement unsharpness squared + screen unsharpness squared]
B. Minimum total unsharpness occurs when the individual blurrings are nearly equal
C. Signal to noise ratio (SNR) is reduced when a large number of x-ray photons are absorbed by a screen
D. The use of screens decreases noise
E. Using a higher kV reduces SNR

QUESTION 13
Computed Tomography (CT)

A. Back projection is more effective than filtered back projection at reducing the blurring at edges of an image
B. Partial volume effects are reduced by using both a large slice thickness and large pixel size
C. Soft tissues, excluding fat, only cover a range of about 80 CT numbers
D. The effect of beam hardening is the progressive reduction in the CT number of an individual tissue as it is traversed by the x-ray beam
E. 'Bow tie' filters are used to compensate for the diminishing patient thickness towards the edges of the fan beam

QUESTION 14
The following statements are true

A. In gamma imaging, spatial resolution (SR) can be calculated from the full width at half maximum (FWHM) of a line source
B. The intrinsic resolution of a gamma camera is 1-2mm
C. Linearity of a gamma camera can be assessed by imaging a flood field source
D. Energy resolution of a gamma camera is typically 25% of the peak energy
E. The better the energy resolution of a gamma camera, the better its spatial resolution

QUESTION 15
The following statements are true

A. Local rules are enforced by the radiation protection supervisor (RPS)
B. Local rules are a legal document
C. The department of the environment is responsible for enforcing the Radioactive Substances Act 1993
D. The Health & Safety Executive (HSE) is responsible for enforcing the IRR 85
E. The Department of the Environment is responsible for enforcing the IRR 88

QUESTION 16
Regarding ultrasound (U/S)

A. Acoustic Impedance = Velocity of U/S in a material divided by the density of the material
B. The intensity of U/S is inversely proportional to the square of the wave amplitude
C. The intensity of U/S is measured in watts per square millimetre
D. The velocity of U/S in air equals 400 metres per second
E. The average velocity of U/S in soft tissue equals 1,000 metres per second

QUESTION 17
Regarding ultrasound (U/S)

A. Real time U/S scanning can be performed with a phased array sector transducer
B. Real time U/S scanning cannot be performed with a stepped linear array transducer
C. Real time U/S scanning can be performed with a mechanical sector scanner
D. In real time scanning, the imaging frame rate is directly related to the pulse repetition frequency (PRF)
E. Increasing the PRF improves the imaging of deep structures

QUESTION 18
Regarding MRI

A. Precessing protons are brought into phase by the application of a radio-frequency (RF) pulse
B. A RF pulse of 10-20 ms is required to "flip" the protons from their precessing state
C. The frequency of the RF generator is most effective if it is matched to the Larmor precession of the dipoles
D. The net magnetic vector in the direction of the external magnetic field is responsible for producing a MR signal
E. The peak MR signal is proportional to the proton density within a voxel

QUESTION 19
Regarding resistive magnets used in MRI

A. Can typically weigh up to 80 tonnes
B. May consume some 50-100 kW of power
C. Can provide field strengths up to 2T
D. Require a large water cooling system
E. Can be switched to stand-by to reduce consumption

QUESTION 20
Regarding flow phenomena in MRI

A. Even-echo rephasing produces signal loss in venous blood
B. Even-echo rephasing only occurs with multi-echo sequences
C. Even-echo rephasing is due to an even number of 180 degree pulses successfully rephasing protons which have been dephased by motion
D. Misregistration artefact is exhibited by vessels passing parallel to the axis of a slice
E. In cerebral T2 weighted imaging, CSF in the cerebral aqueduct produces more signal than that in the ventricles

QUESTION 21
Regarding the basal ganglia

A. The caudate nucleus is highly curved and lies within the concavity of the lateral ventricle
B. The lentiform nucleus is made of a smaller medial globus palladus and larger lateral putamen
C. The claustrum is a thin sheet of white matter and lies between putamen and insula
D. The amygdaloid body is part of the caudate nucleus
E. The globus palladus has a lower signal than surrounding brain in MRI

QUESTION 22
Regarding normal variation

A. A secondary ossification centre may be seen in the supero-lateral aspect of the patella
B. Fibular spurs may be seen below the head of the fibula pointing in a cranial direction
C. A groove on the medial femoral condyle may be caused by popliteus tendon
D. On an AP radiograph the tibial tubercle may cause a lucent area over the tibia
E. On a lateral radiograph a projection on the posterior surface of the tibia may represent the insertion of soleus muscle

QUESTION 23
Concerning the hip joint

A. Gluteus maximus is an extensor
B. The psoas bursa lies between the ilio-femoral ligament and the capsule
C. The nerve to rectus femoris supplies the joint
D. The acetabular labrum is deficient inferiorly and continues as the transverse ligament
E. The pubofemoral ligament attaches to the superior part of the capsule

QUESTION 24
Regarding radiography of the elbow

A. The beam is centred 2.5 cm proximal to the epicondyles in the AP view
B. The posterior fat pad is not usually visible
C. An anterior fat pad indicates a joint effusion
D. Both elbows should be x-rayed when a sole injury is suspected in a child
E. The epiphysis of the radial head appears at 4 years

QUESTION 25
Regarding the scapula

A. The coracoid process projects anteriorly from the upper border
B. The inferior angle usually lies over the seventh rib
C. An ossification centre for the body appears at the eighth intrauterine week
D. It gives a large attachment for subscapularis on its dorsal surface
E. The coracoclavicular ligament is made up of two parts, conoid and trapezoid

QUESTION 26

The prostate gland

A. Has smooth muscle continuous with the bladder
B. Is normally broader than it is long
C. Has a lower surface called the base
D. Lies below the levator ani complex
E. Drains to internal and external iliac nodes

QUESTION 27

In an axial CT image at the level of the hip joints

A. Seminal vesicles are seen posterior to the bladder in the male
B. Sartorius muscle is seen lateral to the tensor fasciae latae
C. The femoral artery lies on pectineus muscle
D. The inferior pubic ramus is seen
E. Rectus femoris muscle is in contact with the greater trochanter of the femur

QUESTION 28

Sites of porto-systemic anastomosis include

A. Lower end of oesophagus
B. Upper part of anal canal
C. Quadrate lobe of liver
D. Periumbilical region
E. Caecum

QUESTION 29

Regarding the anterior abdominal wall

A. The properitoneal fat line is caused by fatty tissue between visceral and parietal peritoneum
B. The properitoneal fat line is absent in approximately 18% of cases
C. External oblique muscle is partially inserted into the linea alba
D. The median umbilical ligament is the remnant of the umbilical artery
E. Transversus abdominis does not insert into the linea alba

QUESTION 30

The portal vein

A. Is formed by the union of inferior mesenteric and splenic veins
B. Is approx. 8 cm long
C. Has the left gastric vein as a tributary
D. Drains the entire gut from lower oesophagus to upper anal canal
E. Ascends posterior to the first part of the duodenum

QUESTION 31

The following statements are true

A. The descending colon has a mesentery in 20% of adults
B. The arteria pancreatica magna is a branch of the splenic artery
C. The liver is developed from foregut
D. The prepyloric vein (of Mayo) drains the first and second parts of the duodenum
E. Ileal arteries form a series of arcades in the mesentery

QUESTION 32

Regarding the spinal cord

A. The conus medullaris lies at the level of L3 at birth
B. The filum terminale is attached to the second sacral vertebra
C. The dorsal and ventral roots unite 2cm beyond the intervertebral foramen to form the spinal nerve
D. The anterior median sulcus is deeper than the posterior median sulcus
E. The central canal extends 5-6mm into the filum terminale

QUESTION 33

The following statements are true

A. The pulmonary trunk divides immediately after leaving the fibrous pericardium
B. The division of the pulmonary trunks is posterior to the left main bronchus
C. The artery for the right upper lobe passes anterior to the right upper lobe bronchus
D. The pulmonary trunk is attached to the aortic arch at its concavity by the ligamentum arteriosum
E. The normal venous pressure of pulmonary vessels is 10mm of mercury

QUESTION 34

The following statements are true

A. The azygous vein enters the superior vena cava on its lateral aspect
B. The SVC has 2-3 valves near its termination
C. The SVC may be left sided in 0.3% of cases
D. The SVC is related immediately to the right phrenic nerve
E. The SVC is formed at level T3/T4

QUESTION 35

The following are true

A. The tuberculum sellae is a constituent of the sphenoid bone
B. The carotid sulci is a constituent of the body of sphenoid bone
C. The trigeminal nerve supplies motor fibres to muscles of mastication
D. The trigeminal nerve arises from the mid brain
E. The trigeminal nerve arises from the posterior surface of the brain stem

QUESTION 36

The following statements are true

- A. The cranial dura matter is in two layers
- B. The falx cerebri is narrower at its posterior attachment
- C. The diaphragma sellae is attached to all four clinoid processes
- D. The sheath of meninges around the optic nerve extends up to the optic canal
- E. The spinal dura matter extends up to the second sacral vertebra

QUESTION 37

Regarding the middle ear

- A. The lateral and medial walls curve inwards and are about 6mm apart in its middle aspect
- B. The cordatympanic nerve passes between the tympanic membrane and the handle of malleus
- C. The epitympanic recess only accommodates the head of malleus and body of incus
- D. The promontory is formed by the second turn of cochlea
- E. The oval window lies below the round window

QUESTION 38

The following are true

- A. The thoracic inlet measures about 15cm wide and 5cm anteroposteriorly
- B. The thoracic inlet is widest from side to side
- C. The body of sternum is formed by four pieces of sternebrae
- D. The transverse crest of the ribs is attached to the intervertebral discs
- E. The subclavius muscle is attached to the inferior surface of the first rib

QUESTION 39

The following statements are true

- A. The incidence of cervical ribs is 1-2%
- B. The accessory hemidiaphragm is more common on the right side
- C. The incidence of bilateral cervical ribs is 5%
- D. The right diaphragm is normally higher than the left by about 2cm
- E. Bony thoracic anomalies are more common in the lower most ribs

QUESTION 40

Regarding the hyoglossus muscle

- A. It is crossed superficially by the lingual nerve
- B. It has the glossopharyngeal nerve deep to it
- C. It is derived from suboccipital myotomes
- D. It protracts the tongue
- E. It has the lingual artery running superficial to it

QUESTION 41
When using ultrasound to image the head and neck

A. The facial nerve can be demonstrated in the parotid gland in 50% of cases
B. Swallowing can improve visualisation of the retrosternal goitre
C. The submental approach is used to ultrasound the base of the tongue
D. Lymph nodes of less than 5 mm in length cannot be accurately detected
E. Ultrasound can be used to visualise the vocal chords

QUESTION 42
During lymphangiography of the lower limb

A. It is normal to see less than 5 vessels entering the inguinal nodes
B. It is normal to see contrast media in the vessels at 24 hours
C. The paraaortic lymph nodes do not normally extend laterally beyond the tips of the transverse processes
D. It is common to see a gap in the chain of lymph nodes at L5 on the right
E. The left supraclavicular glands rarely fill after pedal lymphangiography

QUESTION 43
Regarding lymphoscintigraphy

A. 1-3 mls of ^{99m}Tc-nanocolloid is injected subcutaneously
B. Static images are acquired over 3 hours
C. Complete blockage is indicated by absent lumbo-sacral uptake at 24 hours
D. Ischiorectal injections demonstrate the iliopelvic lymphatics
E. Rib periosteal injections can be used to demonstrate the internal mammary chain

QUESTION 44
Regarding ultrasound of the testicle

A. The tunica albuginea is highly reflective
B. The mediastinum testes is a thin reflective band lying in the short axis of the testis
C. The epididymis is hypoechoic when compared to the testis
D. It is normal to have some free scrotal fluid
E. The rete testis is a small intratesticular tubular structure adjacent to the epididymis

QUESTION 45
When imaging the prostate

A. The seminal vesicles appear as a bow-tie shaped highly echogenic structure on ultrasound
B. The peripheral zone is distinguishable from the transition zone on T1W MRI
C. The peripheral zone is distinguishable from the transitional zone on T2W MRI
D. During transrectal prostate biopsy at least six fine needle aspirate samples should be performed
E. Haematuria is a recognised complication following transrectal ultrasound biopsy of the prostate

QUESTION 46
Regarding micturating cystograms in the infant

A. Prophylactic antibiotics are used
B. Sedation is advisable
C. Contrast media induced cystitis is a recognised complication
D. A 5 French feeding tube is used to catheterise
E. The catheter is rapidly withdrawn during micturation

QUESTION 47
Regarding pelvic sonography

A. A retroverted uterus is demonstrated better by transabdominal than transvaginal scanning
B. Higher frequency transducers are required for transabdominal sonography than transvaginal sonography
C. Transvaginal sonography requires a full bladder
D. Transabdominal sonography requires a full bladder
E. When a full bladder is required, over distention can occur

QUESTION 48
Regarding MIBG scans

A. Myocardial uptake is normal
B. Reserpine can result in a false negative scan
C. Images are acquired at 30 minutes and 3 hours
D. Injection can result in hypertension
E. Amiodorone can result in a false negative scan

QUESTION 49
Regarding oral cholecystography

A. Minor side effects are experienced in 15%
B. Can induce thyrotoxicosis
C. Can induce gout
D. Can precipitate toxicity of protein bound drugs
E. Reliably demonstrates the duct

QUESTION 50
Regarding percutaneous cholangiography

A. Active cholangitis is an absolute contraindication
B. Non-dilatation of the biliary tree is a contraindication
C. Prophylactic antibiotics are required
D. Is contraindicated in hyadatid disease
E. Being unfit for surgery is a relative contraindication

QUESTION 51

Small bowel enema intubation

- A. The catheter may not pass into the duodenum due to coiling in the fundus
- B. Use double-backed manouvre to get out of fundus
- C. Turn patient right side down when using a weighted tip catheter
- D. Inject contrast to outline antrum/duodenum
- E. If difficult to intubate the duodenum, turn patient prone

QUESTION 52

CT of the oesophagus

- A. Positive oral contrast is advised
- B. 2% gastrograffin solution can be used
- C. Prone views are preferable
- D. Maxolon 10 mg IV is routinely administered
- E. CT is imaging modality of choice for staging

QUESTION 53

SMA Angiography

- A. A coeliac angiogram should be performed prior to a sub-angio
- B. Bowel preparation is required
- C. Abdominal compression is required
- D. Arterial phase - 2 films per second for six seconds is appropriate
- E. Venous phase - 1 per second for six seconds is appropriate

QUESTION 54

NIH catheters

- A. Have no end hole
- B. Have no side holes
- C. Are inserted through a sheath
- D. Are excellent selective arterial catheters
- E. Can be used for cerebral angiography

QUESTION 55

Coronary Angiography

- A. Catheterisation of the right main coronary is relatively easier than the left
- B. Left main stem catheterisation is the first study to be performed
- C. LV study is performed to look at left ventricle movement
- D. LV study is performed to look at mitral valve function
- E. An arch aortogram is done to check the aortic valve function

QUESTION 56

The following knee MRI sequences best identify the following structures

A. Sagittal gradient echo - menisci
B. Volume sagittal T2 - medial collateral ligaments
C. Sagittal volume - ACL
D. Axial T1 - medial retinaculum
E. Sagittal volume GE - fibular lateral ligament

QUESTION 57

Radionuclide bone imaging - 3-phase imaging

A. Arterial phase at 1-2 frames per second
B. Arterial phase lasts 5 minutes
C. Blood pool phase images are taken every minute for 3 minutes
D. Blood pool phase is at 5 minutes
E. Delayed views are the same as for static imaging

QUESTION 58

The following are appropriate centering points

A. Trauma obliques - mid clavicle
B. Lateral cervical spine - 2.5 cms inferior to the angle of the mandible
C. Lateral lumbar spine - 2.5 cms anterior to L3 spinous process
D. Odontoid peg - centre of the mouth
E. AP thoracic spine - midway between the manubrium and the xiphisternum

QUESTION 59

The following are true regarding contrast media for bronchography

A. Aqueous Dionosil is appropriate
B. Lipiodol is appropriate
C. Conray 240 is appropriate
D. Non-ionic Dimer is appropriate
E. Iohexol 300 is better than Iotrolan 300

QUESTION 60

The following are centering points are correct

A. Lateral thoracic spine - 2.5 cms anterior to the spinous process of T6
B. AP lumbar spine - midline of the lower costal margin
C. Lateral lumbar spine - 10 cms anterior to the spinous process of L3
D. Right posterior oblique of lumbar spine - lower costal margin in the mid-axillary line
E. Coned lateral of L5/S1 - 7.5 cms anterior to the L5 spinous process

Exam 3: Answers

ANSWER 1
A. TRUE   B. TRUE   C. TRUE   D. TRUE   E. FALSE

As lower exposures are required with fast film screen systems, the use of rarer screens can lead to problems with noise

Ref: Curry & Thomas. Christensen's Physics of Diagnostic Radiology. 4th Edition. Williams and Wilkins (Europe) Ltd.

ANSWER 2
A. FALSE   B. FALSE   C. TRUE   D. FALSE   E. FALSE

The photoelectric effect involves an interaction with a bound electron
A positron is emitted in pair production
Most scatter in diagnostic radiology is produced by the Compton process. However when contrast agents such as barium and iodine are used, secondary radiation via the photoelectric effect may reach the film

Ref: Curry & Thomas. Christensen's Physics of Diagnostic Radiology. 4th Edition. Williams & Wilkins (Europe) Ltd.

ANSWER 3
A. TRUE   B. TRUE   C. TRUE   D. FALSE   E. TRUE

The tube current is measured in mA

Ref: Curry & Thomas. Christensen's Physics of Diagnostic Radiology. 4th Edition. Williams & Wilkins (Europe) Ltd.

ANSWER 4
A. TRUE   B. FALSE   C. FALSE   D. TRUE   E. TRUE

Alpha particles have a relatively large mass and this together with their double charge means that they travel relatively slowly through matter and produce a large amount of ionization per unit length of track

Ref: Armstrong. Lecture Notes on the Physics of Radiology. 1st Edition. 1990. Clinical Press Ltd.

ANSWER 5

A. FALSE   B. FALSE   C. FALSE   D. TRUE   E. TRUE

Lateral decentering produces a uniformly light radiograph

Focus grid distance decentering produces a film which is light at the periphery

Combined lateral and focus grid distance decentering produces a radiograph that is light on one side and dark on the other

There is an increased patient dose incurred with moving grids due to the inevitable lateral decentering that occurs resulting in primary radiation losses of up to 20%

Ref: Armstrong. Lecture Notes on the Physics of Radiology. 1st Edition. 1990. Clinical Press Ltd.

ANSWER 6

A. FALSE   B. TRUE   C. FALSE   D. TRUE   E. FALSE

Narrow angle tomography is otherwise known as zonography

Wide angle tomography is most effective in studying tissues that have a lot of natural contrast i.e. the inner ear. Conversely narrow angled tomography is useful for imaging tissues with low natural contrast, i.e. the kidneys

A phantom image may occur as a result of the superimposition of the blur margins of regularly recurring structures. Alternatively they may also be produced by the displacement of the blur margins of dense objects which then simulate less dense objects

Narrow angled tomography uses a narrow arc and aims to see the whole of a particular structure, undistorted and sharply defined, It is wide angled tomography that utilises maximal blurring

Ref: Armstrong. Lecture Notes on the Physics of Radiology. 1st Edition. 1990. Clinical Press Ltd.

ANSWER 7

A. FALSE   B. TRUE   C. FALSE   D. TRUE   E. TRUE

^{123}I has a half life of 13 hours

^{125}I is a gamma emitter.

^{123}I emits a gamma ray with an energy of 159 KeV

^{131}I emits gamma rays with energies of 80, 204 and 364 KeV

Ref. Curry & Thomas. Christensen's Physics of Diagnostic Radiology. 4th Edition. Williams & Wilkins (Europe) Ltd.

ANSWER 8

A. TRUE   B. TRUE   C. TRUE   D. TRUE   E. TRUE

Inherent film contrast is determined by the size and distribution of the grains of silver halide produced in the manufacturing process

Film fog, in turn, is determined by the way the film is stored and its developing conditions

Subject contrast is influenced by several factors such as KV, scatter radiation, differences in patient thickness, differences in density and atomic number

The way a film is stored and the conditions under which it is developed have an effect on film fog

Ref: Armstrong. Lecture Notes on the Physics of Radiology. 1st Edition. Clinical Press Ltd.

ANSWER 9

A. FALSE   B. FALSE   C. FALSE   D. FALSE   E. FALSE

The average annual total ED to the population is 2.5 mSv

Medical investigations contribute about 14% of the average annual ED

Medical staff, through adequate shielding, should receive very low doses, almost on par with the general population

Potassium-40 is a natural radionuclide in food. The major contributors from the ground are radon and thoron

People in Cornwall receive an annual total ED about three times the national average

Ref: Curry & Thomas. Christensen's Physics of Diagnostic Radiology. 4th Edition. Williams & Wilkins (Europe) Ltd.

ANSWER 10

A. TRUE   B. TRUE   C. FALSE   D. FALSE   E. TRUE

A high energy beam is more penetrating than a low energy beam . Hence an absorber is less efficient at attenuating at high energies

Muscle has a greater physical density than fat and consequently has a higher linear attenuation coefficient

Ref: Curry & Thomas. Christensen's Physics of Diagnostic Radiology. 4th Edition. Williams & Wilkins (Europe) Ltd.

ANSWER 11

A. TRUE   B. FALSE   C. TRUE   D. FALSE   E. FALSE

W is chosen as the target material because of its high Z, high melting point and low vapour pressure

The square of the kVp, mAs, atomic number and waveform determine the number of x-rays produced i.e., the quantity

X-ray production is 1% efficient. 99% of the incident energy goes into heat production

Ref: Farr & Allisy-Roberts. Physics for Medical Imaging. 1st Edition. W B Saunders Co Ltd.

ANSWER 12

A. TRUE   B. TRUE   C. FALSE   D. FALSE   E. TRUE

SNR increases with an increasing number of xray photons absorbed

The use of screens increases noise

However a higher kV also incurs less dose to the patient

Ref: Farr & Allisy-Roberts. Physics for Medical Imaging. 1st Edition. W B Saunders Co Ltd.

ANSWER 13

A. FALSE   B. FALSE   C. TRUE   D. TRUE   E. TRUE

Filtered back projection is more effective at reducing the blurring at edges of an image

Both thinner slices and smaller pixels should be used to reduce partial volume artefacts. Thus making it more likely that high contrast objects are contained within their own voxel, and do not increase the average CT number of neighbouring voxels

Ref: Farr & Allisy-Roberts. Physics for Medical Imaging. 1st Edition. W B Saunders Co Ltd.

ANSWER 14

A. TRUE   B. TRUE   C. FALSE   D. FALSE   E. TRUE

Imaging a line source provides a line spread function from which FWHM is calculated

Linearity is assessed by imaging a line source

Energy resolution is the ability to distinguish between separate gamma rays of differing energies. It is typically 12% of the peak energy

With improved energy resolution there is better resolution of scatter resulting in improved spatial resolution

Ref: Farr & Allisy-Roberts. Physics for Medical Imaging. 1st Edition. W B Saunders Co Ltd.

ANSWER 15

A. FALSE   B. TRUE   C. TRUE   D. TRUE   E. FALSE

The local rules are policed by the RPS, but enforced by the local HSE Inspector

Enforcing the IRR 88 is the responsibility of the Secretary of State for Health who uses the appropriate HSE

Ref: Farr & Allisy-Roberts. Physics for Medical Imaging. 1st Edition. W B Saunders Co Ltd.

ANSWER 16

A. FALSE   B. FALSE   C. TRUE   D. FALSE   E. FALSE

Acoustic impedance = velocity of U/S multiplied by the density of the material

The intensity of U/S is proportional to the square of the wave amplitude

Velocity of U/S in air = 330 metres per second

The average velocity of U/S in soft tissue = 1540 metres per second

Ref: Farr & Allisy-Roberts. Physics for Medical Imaging. 1st Edition. W B Saunders Co Ltd.

ANSWER 17

A. TRUE   B. FALSE   C. TRUE   D. TRUE   E. FALSE

With a stepped linear array transducer, piezoelectric elements are energised in overlapping groups so that the transducer scans a rectangular area of the body

PRF = frame rate x lines per frame

Depth of view is inversely proportional to the PRF

Ref: Farr & Allisy-Roberts. Physics for Medical Imaging. 1st Edition. W B Saunders Co Ltd.

ANSWER 18
A. TRUE   B. FALSE   C. TRUE   D. FALSE   E. TRUE

A RF pulse of 1ms or less is needed to flip the protons from their precessing state

It is the transverse component of the magnetic vector that produces the MR signal

Ref: Farr & Allisy-Roberts. Physics for Medical Imaging. 1st Edition. W B Saunders Co Ltd.

ANSWER 19
A. FALSE   B. TRUE   C. FALSE   D. TRUE   E. TRUE

These are the smallest and "lightest" of the magnets used in MRI, weighing some 2 tonnes. However only low field strengths up to 0.5T are possible.

Ref: Farr & Allisy-Roberts. Physics for Medical Imaging. 1st Edition. W B Saunders Co Ltd.

ANSWER 20
A. FALSE   B. TRUE   C. TRUE   D. FALSE   E. FALSE

Even-echo rephasing produces paradoxical enhancement in veins and in the periphery of arteries where the high signal may mimic a thrombus

Misregistration artefact: Vessels passing obliquely through a slice exhibit this phenomenon - if one considers a sample of blood passing through the imaging plane, some of the sample will remain within the slice long enough to receive both the 90 degree and 180 degree pulses required to produce a spin echo. However, by the time the echo is produced the sample will have moved obliquely out of the imaging plane and so the readout gradient applied at this time will wrongly localise the vessel to the current position of the sample. This may be manifest as a hypo intense circle with the hyper intense blood displaced to one side.

Flow through the cerebral aqueduct is quite fast compared to the ventricles and consequently produces signal loss

Ref: Curry & Thomas. Christensen's Physics of Diagnostic Radiology. 4th Edition. Williams & Wilkins (Europe) Ltd.

ANSWER 21
A. TRUE   B. TRUE   C. FALSE   D. TRUE   E. TRUE

The claustrum is not white matter but a sheet of grey matter

The globus palladus has a lower signal in MRI because of its high iron content.

Refs:
Anatomy for Diagnostic Imaging. Ryan & McNicholas. W B Saunders Co Ltd.
Essential Anatomy by Lumley, Craven & Aitken. 3rd Edition. Churchill Livingstone.
Clinical Anatomy by Harold Ellis. 8th edition. Churchill Livingstone.

ANSWER 22

A. TRUE   B. FALSE   C. FALSE   D. TRUE   E. TRUE

Fibular spurs point in a caudal direction

The lateral condyle is grooved by popliteus tendon

Refs:
Anatomy for Diagnostic Imaging. Ryan & McNicholas. W B Saunders Co Ltd.
Atlas of Normal Roentgen Variants. Keats. 6th Edition. Mosby.

ANSWER 23

A. TRUE   B. FALSE   C. TRUE   D. TRUE   E. FALSE

Psoas bursa lies superficial to the ilio femoral ligament and joint capsule

The pubofemoral ligament attaches to the inferior part of the capsule

Ref: Last's Anatomy. McMinn. 9th Edition. Churchill Livingstone.

ANSWER 24

A. FALSE   B. TRUE   C. FALSE   D. FALSE   E. TRUE

The beam is centred 2.5 cm distal to the epicondyles

An anterior fat pad may be a normal finding

This is not an indication for bilateral x-rays in children

Refs:
Diagnostic Radiography. Bryan. 3rd Edition. Churchill Livingstone.
Anatomy for Diagnostic Imaging. Ryan & McNicholas. W B Saunders Co Ltd.
An Atlas of Anatomy Basic to Radiology. Meschan. W B Saunders Co Ltd.

ANSWER 25

A. TRUE   B. TRUE   C. TRUE   D. FALSE   E. TRUE

Subscapularis attaches to the ventral surface of the scapula

Refs:
Last's Anatomy. McMinn. 9th Edition. Churchill Livingstone.
Anatomy for Diagnostic Imaging. Ryan & McNicholas. W B Saunders Co Ltd.

ANSWER 26

A. TRUE   B. TRUE   C. FALSE   D. FALSE   E. TRUE

The base of the prostate is its upper surface

The prostate lies above the levator ani complex

Refs:
Last's Anatomy. McMinn. 9th Edition. Churchill Livingstone.
Gray's Anatomy. 38th Edition. Churchill Livingstone.

ANSWER 27

A. TRUE   B. FALSE   C. FALSE   D. FALSE   E. FALSE

Sartorius is medial to tensor fasciae lata

The femoral vein lies between the artery and pectineus

The superior pubic ramus can be seen

Rectus femoris is in contact with the head of the femur

Refs:
Last's Anatomy. McMinn. 9th Edition. Churchill Livingstone.
Imaging Atlas of Human Anatomy. Weir & Abrahams. 2nd Edition. Mosby.

ANSWER 28

A. TRUE   B. TRUE   C. FALSE   D. TRUE   E. FALSE

The bare area of the liver is a site of a porto-systemic anastomosis

Other sites of anastomosis include retroperitoneal areas, not the caecum

Refs:
Last's Anatomy. McMinn. 9th Edition. Churchill Livingstone.
Gray's Anatomy. 38th Edition. Churchill Livingstone.

ANSWER 29

A. FALSE   B. TRUE   C. TRUE   D. FALSE   E. FALSE

The properitoneal fat line is caused by fatty tissue between the anterior abdominal wall and peritoneum

The median umbilical ligament is the remnant of the urachus

Transversus abdominis does insert into the linea alba

Refs:
Last's Anatomy. McMinn. 9th Edition. Churchill Livingstone.
Gray's Anatomy. 38th Edition. Churchill Livingstone.
Anatomy for Diagnostic Imaging. Ryan & McNicholas. W B Saunders Co Ltd.

ANSWER 30

A. FALSE   B. TRUE   C. TRUE   D. TRUE   E. TRUE

The portal vein is formed by the union of the superior mesenteric and splenic veins

Refs:
Last's Anatomy. McMinn. 9th Edition. Churchill Livingstone.
Gray's Anatomy. 38th Edition. Churchill Livingstone.

ANSWER 31

A. TRUE   B. TRUE   C. TRUE   D. FALSE   E. TRUE

The prepyloric vein drains the first 2.5 cm of duodenum only

Refs:
Last's Anatomy. McMinn. 9th Edition. Churchill Livingstone.
Anatomy for Diagnostic Imaging. Ryan & McNicholas. W B Saunders Co Ltd.

ANSWER 32

A. TRUE   B. FALSE   C. FALSE   D. TRUE   E. TRUE

The filum terminale is attached to the first coccygeal segment.

The dorsal and ventral roots unite at the intervertebral foramen.

Refs:
Anatomy for Diagnostic Imaging. Ryan & McNicholas. W B Saunders Co Ltd.
Essential Anatomy by Lumley, Craven & Aitken. 3rd Edition. Churchill Livingstone.
Clinical Anatomy by Harold Ellis. 8th edition. Churchill Livingstone.

ANSWER 33

A. TRUE   B. FALSE   C. TRUE   D. FALSE   E. FALSE

The division of the pulmonary trunk is anterior to the left main bronchus.

It is not the pulmonary trunk but the left pulmonary artery which is attached to the aortic arch.

Venous pressure of pulmonary vessels is only 3mm of mercury.

Refs:
Anatomy for Diagnostic Imaging. Ryan & McNicholas. W B Saunders Co Ltd.
Essential Anatomy by Lumley, Craven & Aitken. 3rd Edition. Churchill Livingstone.
Clinical Anatomy by Harold Ellis. 8th edition. Churchill Livingstone.

ANSWER 34

A. FALSE   B. FALSE   C. TRUE   D. TRUE   E. TRUE

Enters at its posterior aspect. The SVC is valveless

Refs:
Anatomy for Diagnostic Imaging. Ryan & McNicholas. W B Saunders Co Ltd.
Essential Anatomy by Lumley, Craven & Aitken. 3rd Edition. Churchill Livingstone.
Clinical Anatomy by Harold Ellis. 8th edition. Churchill Livingstone.

ANSWER 35

A. TRUE   B. TRUE   C. TRUE   D. FALSE   E. FALSE

The trigeminal nerve arises from the pons

The trigeminal nerve arises from the anterior surface of the brain stem

Refs:
Anatomy for Diagnostic Imaging. Ryan & McNicholas. W B Saunders Co Ltd.
Essential Anatomy by Lumley, Craven & Aitken. 3rd Edition. Churchill Livingstone.
Clinical Anatomy by Harold Ellis. 8th edition. Churchill Livingstone.

ANSWER 36
A. TRUE   B. FALSE   C. TRUE   D. FALSE   E. TRUE

The falx cerebri is narrower at its anterior attachment and therefore it has a sickle shape

The sheath of meninges around the optic nerve extends up to the sclera

Refs:
Anatomy for Diagnostic Imaging. Ryan & McNicholas. W B Saunders Co Ltd.
Essential Anatomy by Lumley, Craven & Aitken. 3rd Edition. Churchill Livingstone.
Clinical Anatomy by Harold Ellis. 8th edition. Churchill Livingstone.

ANSWER 37
A. FALSE   B. TRUE   C. TRUE   D. FALSE   E. FALSE

It is only 2mm apart at the middle and 6mm apart at the roof

The promontory is formed by the first turn of cochlea

The oval window lies above the round window

Refs:
Anatomy for Diagnostic Imaging. Ryan & McNicholas. W B Saunders Co Ltd.
Essential Anatomy by Lumley, Craven & Aitken. 3rd Edition. Churchill Livingstone.
Clinical Anatomy by Harold Ellis. 8th edition. Churchill Livingstone.

ANSWER 38
A. FALSE   B. TRUE   C. TRUE   D. TRUE   E. FALSE

The thoracic inlet is only 10cm wide

The subclavius muscle is attached to the superior surface at the anterior end of first rib

Refs:
Anatomy for Diagnostic Imaging. Ryan & McNicholas. W B Saunders Co Ltd.
Essential Anatomy by Lumley, Craven & Aitken. 3rd Edition. Churchill Livingstone.
Clinical Anatomy by Harold Ellis. 8th edition. Churchill Livingstone.

ANSWER 39
A. TRUE   B. TRUE   C. FALSE   D. TRUE   E. FALSE

Incidence of bilateral cervical ribs is 50%

Thoracic anomalies are common in the upper four ribs

Refs:
Anatomy for Diagnostic Imaging. Ryan & McNicholas. W B Saunders Co Ltd.
Essential Anatomy by Lumley, Craven & Aitken. 3rd Edition. Churchill Livingstone.
Clinical Anatomy by Harold Ellis. 8th edition. Churchill Livingstone.

ANSWER 40

A. TRUE B. TRUE C. TRUE D. TRUE E. FALSE

Lingual artery runs deep to hyoglossus

Refs:
Anatomy for Diagnostic Imaging. Ryan & McNicholas. W B Saunders Co Ltd.
Essential Anatomy by Lumley, Craven & Aitken. 3rd Edition. Churchill Livingstone.
Clinical Anatomy by Harold Ellis. 8th edition. Churchill Livingstone.

ANSWER 41

A. FALSE B. TRUE C. TRUE D. FALSE E. TRUE

The facial nerve can be seen in 30% of cases. Lymph nodes of 2 mm or greater in size can be accurately detected

Ref: Grainger & Allison. Diagnostic Radiology. 3rd Edition. Churchill Livingstone.

ANSWER 42

A. FALSE B. FALSE C. TRUE D. TRUE E. TRUE

There are 10-15 vessels entering the inguinal nodes. All contrast media should be intra nodal by 24 hours.

Ref: Grainger & Allison. Diagnostic Radiology. 3rd Edition. Churchill Livingstone.

ANSWER 43

A. FALSE B. TRUE C. TRUE D. TRUE E. TRUE

0.1 to 0.3 mls is injected subcutaneously.

Ref: Chapman & Nakielny. A Guide to Radiological Procedures. 3rd Edition. W B Saunders Co Ltd.

ANSWER 44

A. TRUE B. FALSE C. FALSE D. TRUE E. TRUE

The mediastinum testes lies in the long axis of the testis on the same side as the epididymis and represents condensation of connective tissue. The epidydimis is hyperechoic compared to the testes.

Ref: Grainger & Allison. Diagnostic Radiology. 3rd Edition. Churchill Livingstone.

ANSWER 45

A. FALSE B. FALSE C. TRUE D. FALSE E. TRUE

The seminal vesicles are low echogenicity. No differentiation is possible between the transition zone and the peripheral zone on T1W MRI. The peripheral zone is high signal on T2W sequences. Core biopsies are required with at least an 18 gauge needle.

Ref: Grainger & Allison. Diagnostic Radiology. 3rd Edition. Churchill Livingstone.

ANSWER 46
A. TRUE   B. FALSE   C. TRUE   D. TRUE   E. TRUE

Sedation increases the risk of bladder rupture from overfilling.

Ref: Grainger & Allison. Diagnostic Radiology. 3rd Edition. Churchill Livingstone.

ANSWER 47
A. FALSE   B. FALSE   C. FALSE   D. TRUE   E. TRUE

A retroverted uterus is best demonstrated by transvaginal scanning.

Transabdominal scanning uses 3.5 to 5 MHz. Transvaginal scanning uses 5-7.5 MHz. Resolution is therefore improved with transvaginal scanning but the shorter focal zone means that large pelvic masses can be missed. An empty bladder is required for transvaginal scanning.

Ref: Grainger & Allison. Diagnostic Radiology. 3rd Edition. Churchill Livingstone.

ANSWER 48
A. TRUE   B. TRUE   C. FALSE   D. TRUE   E. FALSE

^{131}I MIBG is imaged at 24 and 48 hours. ^{123}I MIBG is imaged at 4 and 24 hours. Tricyclic antidepressants, beta blockers, and phenylephrine will all cause a FALSE negative scan.

Ref: Grainger & Allison. Diagnostic Radiology. 3rd Edition. Churchill Livingstone.

ANSWER 49
A. FALSE   B. TRUE   C. TRUE   D. TRUE   E. FALSE

Minor side effects occur in 50%. Manufacturers recommend a second dose of contrast media 3-4 hours prior to the study to improve visualisation of the duct.

Ref: Chapman & Nakielny. A Guide to Radiological Procedures. 3rd Edition. W B Saunders Co Ltd.

ANSWER 50
A. FALSE   B. FALSE   C. TRUE   D. TRUE   E. TRUE

Active cholangitis is a relative contraindication, drainage of an infected biliary tree may be life saving. PTC is required in those patients unable to undergo ERCP for example following a Whipple's procedure.

Ref: Chapman & Nakielny. A Guide to Radiological Procedures. 3rd Edition. W B Saunders Co Ltd.

ANSWER 51
A. TRUE   B. TRUE   C. TRUE   D. TRUE   E. TRUE

With weighted tip catheters the patient should be turned right side down.

Ref: Whitehouse & Worthington. Techniques in Diagnostic Imaging. 3rd Edition. Blackwell Science Ltd.

ANSWER 52

A. FALSE   B. TRUE   C. TRUE   D. FALSE   E. TRUE

Water is the preferable contrst media. If positive oral contrast is to be given 2% gastrograffin is appropriate. Supine is alright but prone views are recommended as they pull oesophagus away from the mediastum and aorta. Buscopan should be administered. Endoscopic ultrasound is better for local staging but CT evaluates lungs and liver as well and is therefore initially the imaging modality of choice.

Ref: Grainger & Allison. Diagnostic Imaging. 3rd Edition. Churchill Livingstone.

ANSWER 53

A. FALSE   B. FALSE   C. TRUE   D. TRUE   E. FALSE

Patients should be nil by mouth for four hours. The arterial phase requires 2-3 frames per second for 3-5 seconds. The venous phase should be followed for a total of a 20 seconds.

Ref: Chapman & Nakielny. A Guide to Radiological Procedures. 3rd Edition. W B Saunders Co Ltd.

ANSWER 54

A. TRUE   B. FALSE   C. TRUE   D. FALSE   E. FALSE

No guidewires can be used with NIH catheterss and they have to be inserted through a sheath via the common femoral vein. NIH catheters are pecifially for pulmonary angiography.

Ref: Whitehouse & Worthington. Techniques in Diagnostic Imaging. 3rd Edition. Blackwell Science Ltd.

ANSWER 55

A. FALSE   B. FALSE   C. TRUE   D. TRUE   E. TRUE

The left main coronary artery is much easier to catheterise and hence several catheters may sometimes be necessary to catheterise the right. A left ventriclular study should be performed first. During the LV study the catheter is withdrawn and the pressure drop across the aortic valve can be evaluated and in addition during the arch aortogram reflux through the aortic valve can confirm the presence of aortic incompetence.

Ref: Chapman & Nakielny. A Guide to Radiological Procedures. 3rd Edition. W B Saunders Co Ltd.

ANSWER 56

A. TRUE   B. FALSE   C. TRUE   D. TRUE   E. FALSE

The medial collateral ligaments and the fibular collateral ligaments are best demonstrated on coronal T1 sequences.

Ref: MRI in Orthopaedics and Sports Medicine. Stoller. Lippincott Raven.

ANSWER 57
A. TRUE   B. FALSE   C. FALSE   D. TRUE   E. TRUE

The arterial phase lasts one minute. The blood pool phase images are taken for 1-3 minutes.

Ref: Chapman & Nakielny. A Guide to Radiological Procedures. 3rd Edition. W B Saunders Co Ltd.

ANSWER 58
A. TRUE   B. TRUE   C. FALSE   D. TRUE   E. TRUE

A lateral lumber spine is centered 5 cm anterior to L3 spinous process.

Ref: Bell & Finlay. Basic Radiographic Positioning & Anatomy. 1st Edition. Bailliere Tindall.

ANSWER 59
A. FALSE   B. FALSE   C. FALSE   D. TRUE   E. FALSE

Dionosil is no longer made, although it was more viscous and therefore gave better coating. HOCM is extremely dangerous as it can cause severe pulmonary oedema when aspirated. Iotrolan is a new non-ionic dimer agent specifically recommended for bronchography.

Ref: Chapman & Nakielny. A Guide to Radiological Procedures. 3rd Edition. W B Saunders Co Ltd.

ANSWER 60
A. FALSE   B. TRUE   C. TRUE   D. FALSE   E. TRUE

Lateral thoracic spine - 5cms anterior to the spinous process of T6

Right posterior oblique of the lumbar spine - Midclavicular line at the level of the lower costal margin on the raised side

Bell and Finlay. Basic Radiographic Positioning and Anatomy. 1st Edition. Bailliere Tindall.

Exam 4

QUESTION 1

The effects of quantum mottle are reduced by the following

A. When image contrast is high
B. When imaging larger objects
C. By increasing the window width of a digital image
D. By the use of frame averaging in digital subtraction techniques
E. By increasing the kVp when using a film screen combination

QUESTION 2

Regarding x-ray filters

A. Aluminium and Copper are the materials of choice in a compound filter
B. In a compound filter the lower atomic number filter faces the x-ray tube
C. Characteristic radiation produced in the aluminium filter significantly adds to patient skin dose
D. Filtration if the process of decreasing the mean energy of polychromatic radiation by passing it through an absorber
E. The copper in a compound filter is better for dealing with low energy radiation

QUESTION 3

Regarding the production of x-rays

A. Materials of higher atomic number are more efficient x-ray producers
B. Higher energy characteristic radiation is produced with higher atomic number elements
C. The quality of an x-ray beam depends on the square of the kVp
D. The quantity of x-rays produced depends on the mAs
E. Tungsten is commonly used as the anode target material due to its high vapour pressure

QUESTION 4

Regarding the modulation transfer function (MTF)

A. The MTF is calculated from the line spread function by Fourier transformation
B. The total MTF of a complete imaging system is obtained by adding the individual MTF's of each component
C. The frequency of line pairs per mm giving a 10% response on the MTF curve defines the resolving power of an imaging system
D. The maximum value of MTF is normally less than 1
E. MTF is proportional to the ratio of information recorded to the information available

QUESTION 5

Regarding simultaneous multiplane tomography

A. Several layers of x-ray film are all exposed simultaneously during a single tomographic sweep
B. Intensifying screens, of increasing speed, are used between each successive layer of film
C. The reduction in patient dose by using this technique compared to single film tomography is approximately 90%
D. The image quality produced is on par with that of single film tomography
E. The several layers of x-ray film are placed in a special "book cassette" prior to exposure

QUESTION 6

^{131}Iodine has a half life of eight days. Its activity at 9 am on 1st March was 44.4 MBq. Which of the following statements are true regarding the activity after time n, where n equals the number of half lives

A. Activity can be calculated from the formula $A^n = A^o/2^n$, where A^n = decayed activity and A^o = initial activity
B. Its activity at 9 am on 25th March will be 15.5 MBq
C. Its activity at 9 am on 25th March will be 11.1 MBq
D. Its activity at 9 am on 25th March will be 5.55 MBq
E. Its activity at 9 am on 25th March cannot be calculated from the amount of information given

QUESTION 7

Regarding interactions of xray with matter

A. Attenuation = absorption + scatter
B. Half value layer (HVL) is a measure of the penetrating power of an x-ray beam
C. 10 HVLs reduces the intensity of an x-ray beam by a factor of 10
D. Linear attenuation coefficient (LAC) increases as the density of the absorber material increases
E. HVL increases as the density of the absorber increases

QUESTION 8

The following are true

A. Increasing kV reduces the skin dose to the patient
B. Increasing kV reduces the dose to deeper tissues
C. Increasing the focus to film distance (FFD) reduces patient dose
D. The entrance dose for a PA chest x-ray is greater than that of an AP abdominal x-ray
E. Skin dose increases exponentially with increasing mAs

QUESTION 9

Secondary radiation grids

A. Grid cut-off is greatest with both high ratio grids and short grid focus distances
B. With a focused grid, about 50% of the primary radiation is attenuated by the edges of the lead strips
C. Lateral grid decentering produces a uniformly dark film
D. Combined lateral and focus-grid distance decentering produces a radiograph that is light on one side and dark on the other
E. Grids are routinely used when x-raying children

QUESTION 10

The following are true regarding an x-ray tube

A. At the target of an x-ray tube, the effective "focal area" is smaller than the actual "focal area"
B. The target angle is commonly 6-20 degrees
C. An x-ray tube for most diagnostic imaging has 2 filaments and 2 focal spots of differing sizes
D. The effective "focal spot" may be measured with a STAR test tool
E. "Blooming" of a focal spot occurs particularly at low kV values and with small focal spots

QUESTION 11

Regarding films and screens

A. Rare earth screens are faster than calcium tungstate (CaW) screens
B. CaW deliver a patient dose 2-3 times lower than rare earh screens
C. Gadolinium oxysulphide screens may be used with any type of x-ray film
D. Lanthanum oxybromide may be used with ordinary x-ray film
E. The sensitivity of a film may be extended by coating the silver halide crystals with appropriate dyes

QUESTION 12

The following statements regarding the high kV technique are true

A. Subject contrast is high
B. Skin dose is increased
C. Dose to deeper tissues is reduced
D. Grids are less effective compared to use with lower kV techniques
E. Efficiency of x-ray production is low

QUESTION 13
Regarding the image intensifier

A. Brightness gain is the ratio of :- (brightness of the output phosphor : brightness of the input phosphor)
B. Overall brightness gain is typically 5,000-10,000
C. An image is intensified, magnified and inverted by an electron lens
D. Conversion factor is a ratio of :- (luminescence of the output phosphor : input phosphor dose rate)
E. The image produced is uniformly bright and sharp

QUESTION 14
Computed tomography (CT)

A. Second generation scanners are of the translate-rotate type
B. Third generation scanners are of the rotate-rotate type
C. Fourth generation scanners are of the rotate-rotate type
D. Ring artefacts are common with the fourth generation scanner
E. Slip-ring technology has allowed the advent of helical scanning

QUESTION 15
The following statements are true

A. Human error resulting in serious patient over-exposure should be investigated by the Department of Health
B. Equipment fault causing a patient over-exposure greater than twice the dose intended, results in the equipment being withdrawn from use
C. The Department of Health should always be informed of equipment failures
D. It is not necessary to retain the completed request form after an x-ray has been taken
E. The Department of Health recommends that films and other records be kept for a minimum of 6 years

QUESTION 16
Regarding ultrasound (U/S)

A. In continuous mode U/S, the transducer emits a sound of single frequency
B. In pulsed mode U/S, the transducer emits sound with a range of frequencies in a continuous spectrum
C. Quality factor, Q, is the ratio of :- [mean frequency of the ultrasound wave : bandwidth of the transducer]
D. The greater the Quality factor, Q, the narrower the bandwidth of the transducer
E. A transducer with a high Q produces short pulses, and responds to a wide range of frequencies

QUESTION 17
Regarding ultrasound (U/S)

A. Axial resolution deteriorates as the spatial pulse length decreases
B. The higher the frequency of U/S the better the axial resolution
C. Near field lateral resolution improves by the use of a larger transducer
D. A 15 MHz transducer is appropriate for imaging the eye
E. A 3.5 MHz transducer is best suited for examining the thyroid gland

QUESTION 18
Regarding MRI

A. In a spin echo (SE) sequence: the longer the time to echo (TE) the greater the MR signal
B. The greater the spin density (proton density) of a tissue, the larger the MR signal
C. For T1 weighted images, a time to repetition (TR) of 1,000-3,000 ms may be used
D. For T2 weighted images, a TR of 300-800 ms may be used
E. For T1 weighted images, a short TE (30 ms) is used to reduce the effect of T2 on contrast

QUESTION 19
Regarding magnets used in MRI

A. The higher the field strength, the lower the signal to noise ratio
B. The production of an uniform static magnetic field is more difficult with higher field strength magnets
C. Chemical shift artefacts are increased with higher field strength magnets
D. Motion and susceptibility artefacts are worsened with high field strength magnets
E. The fringe field is reduced with higher field strength magnets

QUESTION 20
Regarding MRI artefacts

A. The magic angle phenomenon occurs when a tendon is orientated at 55 degrees to the static magnetic field
B. Titanium produces large signal voids when placed within a static magnetic field
C. Steel produces less signal dropout compared to Titanium
D. Radio frequency interference is usually manifest as a line in the frequency encoding direction
E. Image shading is seen with the use of surface coils

QUESTION 21
The following statements are true

A. The largest white matter association fibres are the corpus callosum
B. The body of corpus callosum lies below the free edge of falx cerebri
C. Splenium is the thickened anterior end of corpus callosum
D. The posterior limb of internal capsule lies between lentiform nucleus and thalamus
E. The posterior most fibres of the internal capsule are occupied by auditory fibres

QUESTION 22

The superficial inguinal lymph nodes receive lymph from

A. Cervix
B. Buttock
C. Testis
D. Umbilicus
E. Glans penis

QUESTION 23

Muscles directly related to the capsule of the hip joint include

A. Piriformis
B. Pectineus
C. Gluteus medius
D. Rectus femoris
E. Quadratus femoris

QUESTION 24

In the upper limb

A. The axillary artery has one branch in its first part
B. The ulnar artery gives rise to the superficial palmar arch
C. The short head of biceps arises from the coracoid process
D. The axillary nerve is damaged in 5% of shoulder dislocations
E. The glenoid labrum is made of hyaline cartilage

QUESTION 25

Regarding the hand

A. A single sesamoid bone is usually seen anterior to the 5th metacarpo-phalangeal joint
B. The first metacarpal has a styloid process on its dorsal aspect
C. The tendons of extensor digitorum insert into the bases of proximal, middle and distal phalanges
D. The shafts of all the phalanges are ossified in utero
E. Secondary ossification centres for all the metacarpals are at the distal ends

QUESTION 26

The following statements are true

A. The sacroiliac joint (SIJ) is a primary cartilaginous joint
B. The sacrotuberous ligament is attached to the transverse tubercles of the sacrum
C. The sacrospinous ligament becomes broader as it passes laterally
D. The sacrococcygeal joint is a symphysis
E. The iliolumbar ligament is attached to the L5 transverse process

QUESTION 27

Regarding the bony pelvis

A. The subpubic angle is greater in females
B. The sacrococcygeal joint is a typical synovial joint
C. Ossification centres for ilium, ischium and pubis all appear before birth
D. The lesser sciatic notch lies above the ischial spine
E. The pubis ossifies in membrane

QUESTION 28

Psoas major muscle

A. Is attached to the transverse processes of the lumbar vertebrae
B. Inserts into the greater trochanter of the femur
C. Is related anteriorly to the lumbar arteries
D. Is related anteriorly to the gonadal arteries on both sides
E. Passes beneath the inguinal ligament

QUESTION 29

Regarding the blood supply of the stomach

A. The right gastric artery supplies the lesser curve
B. The gastroduodenal artery supplies the lesser curve
C. The left gastric artery supplies the greater curve
D. The right gastroepiploic artery is a branch of the gastroduodenal artery
E. Short gastric arteries arise from the left gastroepiploic artery to supply the fundus

QUESTION 30

The common bile duct (CBD)

A. Is approx. 8 cm long
B. Lies in the free edge of the lesser omentum
C. May run through the pancreatic head
D. Lies anterior to the IVC in its middle third
E. Joins the pancreatic duct at an angle of about 90 degrees

QUESTION 31

The ureter

A. On the right is anterior to the third part of the duodenum
B. Is supplied by the common iliac artery
C. Has the gonadal artery posterior to it
D. On the left lies posterior to the left colic artery
E. Is 25 cm long

QUESTION 32

The following statements are true

A. The venous drainage of vertebral column is by valveless veins
B. The conus lies at the level of T12 vertebra at birth
C. The spinal cord is elliptical in cross section with its greater diameter from front to back
D. The anterior median sulcus contains a pair of anterior spinal arteries
E. On a lateral view of the facet joint the cavity is S-shaped

QUESTION 33

The following are true

A. The pulmonary veins enter the mediastinum anterior to the pulmonary arteries
B. The pulmonary veins on the left often unite and enter the left atrium as a single vessel
C. The bronchial arteries arise from the thoracic aorta in 50% of cases
D. There are usually two left and one right bronchial artery
E. The bronchial arteries arise from thoracic aorta at level T10 in 80% of cases

QUESTION 34

Regarding the oesophagus

A. It begins at the level of the upper border of cricoid cartilage
B. Its length is approximately 40cm
C. It inclines to the left at the neck and upper mediastinum and returns to midline at level of T8
D. It traverses the diaphragm at the level of T10
E. Below the level of T4 the azygous vein lies behind and to the right of the oesophagus

QUESTION 35

The following are true

A. The artery of heubner is a branch of middle cerebral artery
B. The posterior choroidal artery is a branch of posterior cerebral artery
C. The pericallosal artery is a branch of anterior cerebral artery
D. The lenticulostriate artery is a branch of middle cerebral artery
E. The anterior choroidal artery is a branch of internal carotid artery

QUESTION 36

The following statements are true

A. The ligamentum denticulatum arises from the pia matter
B. The pia matter lies on the ependymal lining of the ventricles over the roof of the third and fourth ventricles
C. The subarachnoid space is narrowest over the cerebral hemispheres
D. The cisterna magna lies in the angle between the medulla and the cerebellum
E. The subarchnoid space extends along the bundles of olfactory nerves which pierce the cribriform plate

QUESTION 37

Regarding the middle ear

- A. The oval window is closed by the footplate of stapes
- B. The round window is closed by a fibrous disc
- C. The tensor tympani tendon is attached to the body of incus
- D. The auditory tube opens via the medial wall inferiorly
- E. The tegmen tympani separates the middle ear cavity from the anterior cranial fossa

QUESTION 38

The following joints are of the synovial type in the thoracic cage

- A. Costovertebral joints
- B. Costotransverse joints
- C. Manubriosternal joints
- D. Costochondral joint between first costal cartilage and sternum
- E. Costochondral joints between second to seventh costal cartilage and sternum

QUESTION 39

Regarding the fissures of the lung

- A. The minor fissure is seen in 50% of chest xrays
- B. The inferior accessory fissure is seen in 1% of PA chest xrays
- C. The superior accessory fissure is seen in 5% of PA chest xrays
- D. The left transverse fissure is seen in 20% of chest xrays
- E. The azygous fissure is seen in 0.4% of chest xrays

QUESTION 40

The lateral pterygoid muscle

- A. Has the maxillary artery running between its upper and lower heads
- B. It acts as a muscle pump
- C. It is essential for active opening of the mouth
- D. It is supplied by the posterior division of the mandibular nerve
- E. It is embraced by the two heads of the medial pterygoid

QUESTION 41

Regarding lymphangiography

- A. The maximum dose of lipiodol for a 70 kg adult is 7 mls per side
- B. Cytotoxic treatment in the past 3 weeks is a contraindication
- C. The thoracic duct is not usually visualised until 24 hours after injection
- D. The maximum reduction in Tco (carbon monoxide diffusion capacity) occurs in 12 hours
- E. Some dermal backflow is normal

QUESTION 42

Regarding Gallium 67 scanning

A. ⁶⁷Ga-citrate is taken up by normal nasal sinuses
B. ⁶⁷Ga-citrate is taken up by bowel less than ¹¹¹Indium labelled leukocytes
C. ⁶⁷Ga-citrate is given as an IV injection
D. Laxatives are given for two days prior to injection
E. ⁶⁷Ga-citrate emits gamma rays at three principal energies

QUESTION 43

Regarding ultrasound of the peripheral venous system

A. A 3-5 MHz probe is appropriate for superficial veins
B. Venous flow velocity in the arms decreases during inspiration
C. The superficial femoral vein lies postero-medial to the artery
D. The deep veins of the calf are more prominent with the leg elevated
E. The popliteal vein is deep to the artery

QUESTION 44

Regarding ultrasound of the kidneys in a neonate

A. The renal cortex is thin and more reflective than the liver
B. The pyramids may appear large and hypoechoic
C. The normal bladder wall thickness when empty is 1 cm regardless of age
D. The kidneys are best assessed in the prone position
E. Renal length increases by 2 mm for every week of gestation in the fetus

QUESTION 45

An antegrade pyelogram

A. Is contraindicated in ureteral diversion
B. Is contraindicated in renal hyadatid disease
C. Arteriovenous fistulae are a recognised complication
D. Pneumothorax is a recognised complication
E. Macroscopic haematuria is seen in 30% of cases

QUESTION 46

On a submento-vertical projection the following can be seen

A. The foramen rotundum
B. The odontoid peg
C. The foramen rotundum
D. The foramen spinosum
E. The lamdoid suture

QUESTION 47

Regarding ultrasound of the adrenal glands

A. The left are more commonly visualised than the right
B. The adrenal cortex and medulla can be easily differentiated
C. An adrenal gland may be simulated by an accessory spleen
D. An adrenal gland may be simulated by the crux of the diaphragm
E. An adrenal gland may be simulated by a retroperitoneal lymph node

QUESTION 48

The following statements are true of Technetium 99m labelled iminodiacetic acid analogue liver scans

A. A recent meal can result in a false-positive scan
B. An accessory cystic duct can result in a false-positive scan
C. Previous cholecystectomy results in a false-positive scan
D. Acalculous cholecystitis can result in a false-positive scan
E. A duodenal diverticulum can result in a false-positive scan

QUESTION 49

Regarding direct cholangiography

A. In the prone position, the right intrahepatic ducts fill preferentially
B. In the supine position, the right intrahepatic ducts fill preferentially
C. In the supine position the distal common bile duct often fails to opacify
D. Excessive injection can precipitate sepsis
E. 240 mg I /ml is an appropriate concentration

QUESTION 50

The following are true of endoscopic retrograde cholangio-pancreatography

A. Retrograde cholangiography is easier than pancreatography
B. A side viewing endoscope is required
C. Pancreatitic pseudocysts are a contraindication
D. The "trickle" artefact is seen on removing the cannular
E. The presence of oesophageal varices is a contraindication

QUESTION 51

Small bowel enema

A. Maximum normal jejunal calibre is less than 5.5 cms
B. Proximal ileum calibre is usually less than 4 cm
C. Distal ileum calibre less than 3.5 cm
D. 0.5% aqueous solution of Methylcellulose can be helpful
E. Head of single contrast gives better detail than double contrast

QUESTION 52

CT Pneumocolon

A. 10 mm sections advised
B. Rectal contrast is necessary
C. IV Maxolon 10 mg IV is routinely administered
D. No IV contrast is necessary
E. Full bowel preparation is essential

QUESTION 53

Dilatation of oesophagus - technique

A. The pharynx should be anaesthetised first
B. A floppy guidewire should be passed first
C. Catheters are contraindicated
D. The largest balloon available should be used first
E. Angioplasty balloons are helpful

QUESTION 54

Vascular sheaths

A. Have sidearms
B. Have sideholes
C. Should be used for multiple catheter exchanges
D. Should not be used for thrombolysis
E. Should not be used for angioplasty

QUESTION 55

IVC Filter insertion

A. Always use a sheath
B. Always do a venogram first
C. IVC diameter should be at least 3 cms
D. Temporary caval filters should not be left in for more than 12-14 days
E. A birds nest should always be available

QUESTION 56

MRI sequences to look at the triangular fibrocartilage complex (TFCC) of the wrist include

A. Coronal T1
B. Coronal T2
C. Sagittal T1
D. Sagittal STIR
E. Axial T2

QUESTION 57

Regarding radionuclide bone scans

A. Time activity curves are created from blood pool phase
B. Routine tomographic reconstructed images are obtained
C. There is good contrast between bone and soft tissues
D. Renal function can be estimated
E. Complications of this procedure should be explained carefully to the patient

QUESTION 58

Regarding centering points

A. AP hips - 2.5 cms above pubic symphysis
B. AP pelvis - 5 cms above pubic symphysis
C. Lateral ankle - 2.5 cms above medial malleolus
D. AP ankle - midway between medial and lateral malleolus
E. AP foot - midway of 3rd metatarsal shaft

QUESTION 59

Bronchography

A. A lateral view of the left lung is performed
B. A frontal view of the right lung is performed
C. An oblique view of the right lung is performed
D. The right lung should be imaged before the left
E. Spot views are not taken routinely

QUESTION 60

Lung Biopsy can be performed under

A. Single plane screening
B. Biplane screening
C. CT
D. Ultrasound
E. C-arm screening

Exam 4: Answers

ANSWER 1
A. TRUE   B. TRUE   C. FALSE   D. TRUE   E. FALSE

A narrow window width increases image contrast

When using a higher kVp with a film screen combination, the intensification factor of the screen is increased. As a consequence the number of photons required to produce an image is reduced. This results in increased quantum mottle.

Ref: Curry & Thomas. Christensen's Physics of Diagnostic Radiology. 4th Edition. Williams and Wilkins (Europe) Ltd.

ANSWER 2
A. TRUE   B. FALSE   C. FALSE   D. FALSE   E. FALSE

When using a compound filter the higher atomic number material filter (Copper) faces the x-ray tube and the lower atomic number material filter (Aluminium) faces the patient. The purpose of the lower atomic number material is to absorb any characteristic radiation produced in the higher atomic number material

The characteristic radiation produced by the aluminium filter has only a very low energy (1.5 KeV) and is absorbed in the air gap between the patient and the filter

Filtration increases the mean energy of polychromatic radiation

Copper is better for dealing with high energy radiation

Ref: Curry & Thomas. Christensen's Physics of Diagnostic Radiology. 4th Edition. Williams & Wilkins (Europe) Ltd.

ANSWER 3
A. TRUE   B. TRUE   C. FALSE   D. TRUE   E. FALSE

The nature of the target material also determines the energy of the characteristic radiation produced. This is higher for higher atomic number elements

The quality of x-rays depends upon kVp and the waveform. The quantity of x-rays produced depends on the mAs, atomic number, square of the kVp and the waveform

Tungsten has a low vapour pressure in association with a high melting point

Ref: Armstrong: Lecture Notes on the Physics of Radiology. 1st Edition. 1990. Clinical Press Ltd.

ANSWER 4
A. TRUE   B. FALSE   C. TRUE   D. TRUE   E. TRUE

The MTF of a complete system is a product of the individual MTF's of each component

Whilst the MTF is normally less than 1, in xeroradiography values slightly greater than 1 (e.g. 1.1) may be obtained. This is due to the special property in xeroradiography known as edge enhancement

Ref: Armstrong. Lecture Notes on the Physics of Radiology. 1st Edition 1990. Clinical Press Ltd.

ANSWER 5

A. TRUE   B. TRUE   C. FALSE   D. FALSE   E. TRUE

The screens of increasing speed are to allow for the attenuation caused by the reducing intensity of x-rays as they pass through successive layers

The reduction in patient dose is not as great as might be anticipated.

Overall there is an exposure dose per film of about 50% that of single film techniques

This technique results in poor quality tomograms. This is due to the uncontrolled scatter radiation produced which impairs film quality.

Ref: Armstrong. Lecture Notes on the Physics of Radiology. 1st Edition 1990. Clinical Press Ltd.

ANSWER 6

A. TRUE   B. FALSE   C. FALSE   D. TRUE   E. FALSE

Ref: Curry & Thomas. Christensen's Physics of Diagnostic Radiology. 4th Edition. Williams & Wilkins (Europe) Ltd.

ANSWER 7

A. TRUE   B. TRUE   C. FALSE   D. TRUE   E. FALSE

10 HVLs would reduce the intensity by $2^{10} = 1000$

As the density of the absorbing material increases the HVL decreases. HVL is inversely proportional to LAC.

Ref: Farr & Allisy-Roberts. Physics for Medical Imaging. 1st Edition. W B Saunders Co Ltd.

ANSWER 8

A. TRUE   B. TRUE   C. TRUE   D. FALSE   E. FALSE

The entrance dose for a PA chest x-ray = 0.3 mGy: AP abdomen = 10 mGy

Skin dose increases linearly with increasing mAs

Ref: Farr & Allisy-Roberts. Physics for Medical Imaging. 1st Edition. W B Saunders Co Ltd.

ANSWER 9

A. TRUE   B. FALSE   C. FALSE   D. TRUE   E. FALSE

20% of the primary radiation is attenuated by the edges of the lead strips

Lateral grid decentering produces a uniformly light film

Grids are also not used with thin body parts

Ref: Farr & Allisy-Roberts. Physics for Medical Imaging. 1st Edition. W B Saunders Co Ltd.

ANSWER 10

A. TRUE   B. TRUE   C. TRUE   D. TRUE   E. TRUE

Blooming also tends to occur when the tube is operated at high mA as focusing is less precise

Ref: Farr & Allisy-Roberts. Physics for Medical Imaging. 1st Edition. W B Saunders Co Ltd.

ANSWER 11

A. TRUE   B. FALSE   C. FALSE   D. TRUE   E. TRUE

Increased sensitivity of the rare earth phosphors results increased speed compared to CaW screens

Rare earth screens deliver a patient dose 2-3 times lower than CaW screens

Gadolinium oxysulphide may only be used with orthochromatic film (i.e. one sensitive to green light)

Lanthanum oxybromide emits a line spectrum of blue light and hence can be used with ordinary x-ray film which is sensitive to U-V and blue light

Ref: Farr & Allisy-Roberts. Physics for Medical Imaging. 1st Edition. W B Saunders Co Ltd.

ANSWER 12

A. FALSE   B. FALSE   C. TRUE   D. TRUE   E. FALSE

Subject contrast is low

Skin dose is reduced

The amount of scattered radiation is relatively high, thus making grids less effective. Hence the air gap technique is generally preferred.

Efficiency of x-ray production is high and hence there is decreased heat loading which allows very short exposure times.

Ref: Farr & Allisy-Roberts. Physics for Medical Imaging. 1st Edition. W B Saunders Co Ltd.

ANSWER 13

A. TRUE   B. TRUE   C. FALSE   D. TRUE   E. FALSE

The image is minified

The edges of an image are less bright, less sharp and more distorted, due to difficulty of the electron lens in controlling the peripheral electrons. This is known as vignetting.

Ref: Farr & Allisy-Roberts. Physics for Medical Imaging. 1st Edition. W B Saunders Co Ltd.

ANSWER 14

A. TRUE   B. TRUE   C. FALSE   D. FALSE   E. TRUE

Second generation: a narrow fan beam falling on a small curved array of detectors

Third generation: both the beam and detectors rotate

Fourth generation: these are of the rotate-still type. The x-ray tube alone rotates with a stationary ring of detectors

Ring artefacts are most common in third generation scanners

Ref: Farr & Allisy-Roberts. Physics for Medical Imaging. 1st Edition. W B Saunders Co Ltd.

ANSWER 15
A. TRUE   B. FALSE   C. TRUE   D. FALSE   E. TRUE

If the over exposure is greater than 3 times the dose intended, the equipment should be withdrawn. Nevertheless all faults should be investigated and rectified

The DoH should always be informed so that hazard warning notices can be issued nationally as appropriate

A completed request form, signed by a medical practitioner, is a legal document and should be retained, often in the xray packet

Films and records should be kept for 6 years for possible future litigation and for calculations of total patient dose

Ref: Farr & Allisy-Roberts. Physics for Medical Imaging. 1st Edition. W B Saunders Co Ltd.

ANSWER 16
A. TRUE   B. TRUE   C. TRUE   D. TRUE   E. FALSE

A transducer with a high Q produces a pure note and responds only to that note

Ref: Farr & Allisy-Roberts. Physics for Medical Imaging. 1st Edition. W B Saunders Co Ltd.

ANSWER 17
A. FALSE   B. TRUE   C. FALSE   D. TRUE   E. FALSE

The shorter the spatial pulse length, the better the axial resolution

The use of both a smaller transducer and focusing, improve near field lateral resolution

A 7.5 MHz transducer is appropriate for examining the thyroid gland

Ref: Farr & Allisy-Roberts. Physics for Medical Imaging. 1st Edition. W B Saunders Co Ltd.

ANSWER 18
A. FALSE   B. TRUE   C. FALSE   D. FALSE   E. TRUE

SE: The longer the TE, the smaller the MR signal

T1W: short TR: 300-800 ms

T2W: long TR: 1,000-3,000 ms

Ref: Farr & Allisy-Roberts. Physics for Medical Imaging. 1st Edition. W B Saunders Co Ltd.

ANSWER 19
A. FALSE   B. TRUE   C. TRUE   D. TRUE   E. FALSE

Higher field strength magnets provide improved signal to noise ratio

Motion and susceptibility artefacts are worsened due to an increased T1, necessitating a long TR and imaging time, associated with the high field strengths

High field strength magnets are associated with a stronger fringe field

Ref: Farr & Allisy-Roberts. Physics for Medical Imaging. 1st Edition. W B Saunders Co Ltd.

ANSWER 20
A. TRUE   B. FALSE   C. FALSE   D. FALSE   E. TRUE

Tendons are composed of collagen microfibrils which are all orientated in the same direction. Because of this, the physical properties of tendons differ depending on the direction of measurement. The T2 value of tendons is short when they are parallel or perpendicular to the static magnetic field. 55 degrees is the so called magic angle, and the consequence of the magic angle effect is that healthy tendons, while normally of low signal on all sequences, can acquire high signal if orientated at 55 degrees to the static magnetic field. This may mimic tendinous degeneration, tendonitis and tears. This effect only occurs with sequences that employ a relatively short TE. The effect is most likely to be seen in tendons which are curved e.g. supraspinatus tendon.

Titanium is non-ferromagnetic, and has much less marked effect on signal compared to ferromagnetic objects. In fact, small non-ferromagnetic metal objects may be completely missed on MR.

Steel is ferromagnetic. Titanium is non-ferromagnetic.

Radio frequency interference is usually manifest as a line perpendicular to the frequency encoding direction i.e. in the phase encoding direction.

Image shading results from field inhomogeneities. This may produce areas of increased or decreased signal intensity. Regions close to the surface coil appear of higher signal intensity than those further away.

Ref: Curry & Thomas. Christensen's Physics of Diagnostic Radiology. 4th Edition. Williams & Wilkins (Europe) Ltd.

ANSWER 21
A. FALSE   B. TRUE   C. FALSE   D. TRUE   E. TRUE

Corpus callosum is white matter fibres of commissural type

Splenium is the thickened posterior end of the corpus callosum.

Refs:
Anatomy for Diagnostic Imaging. Ryan & McNicholas. W B Saunders Co Ltd.
Essential Anatomy by Lumley, Craven & Aitken. 3rd Edition. Churchill Livingstone.
Clinical Anatomy by Harold Ellis. 8th edition. Churchill Livingstone.

ANSWER 22
A. FALSE   B. TRUE   C. FALSE   D. TRUE   E. FALSE

The cervix drains to external and internal iliac nodes

The testis drains to para aortic nodes

The glans penis drains to deep inguinal nodes

Refs:
Last's Anatomy. McMinn. 9th Edition. Churchill Livingstone.
Gray's Anatomy. 38th Edition. Churchill Livingstone.

ANSWER 23

A. TRUE   B. TRUE   C. FALSE   D. TRUE   E. FALSE

Gluteus minimus lies between gluteus medius and the hip joint

Obturator externus lies between quadratus femoris and the hip joint

Ref: Last's Anatomy. McMinn. 9th Edition. Churchill Livingstone.

ANSWER 24

A. TRUE   B. TRUE   C. TRUE   D. TRUE   E. FALSE

The labrum is made of fibrocartilage

Refs:
Last's Anatomy. McMinn. 9th Edition. Churchill Livingstone.
Anatomy for Diagnostic Imaging. Ryan & McNicholas. W B Saunders Co Ltd.

ANSWER 25

A. TRUE   B. TRUE   C. TRUE   D. TRUE   E. FALSE

The secondary ossification centre for the thumb metacarpal is at its proximal end

Refs:
Last's Anatomy. McMinn. 9th Edition. Churchill Livingstone.
Anatomy for Diagnostic Imaging. Ryan & McNicholas. W B Saunders Co Ltd.

ANSWER 26

A. FALSE   B. TRUE   C. FALSE   D. TRUE   E. TRUE

The SIJ is an atypical synovial joint

The sacrospinous ligament narrows as it passes laterally

Refs:
Last's Anatomy. McMinn. 9th Edition. Churchill Livingstone.
Gray's Anatomy. 38th Edition. Churchill Livingstone.

ANSWER 27

A. TRUE   B. FALSE   C. TRUE   D. FALSE   E. FALSE

The sacrococcygeal joint is a symphysis

The lesser sciatic notch lies between the ischial spine and tuberosity

The pubis ossifies in cartilage

Ref: Last's Anatomy. McMinn. 9th Edition. Churchill Livingstone.

ANSWER 28

A. TRUE   B. FALSE   C. FALSE   D. TRUE   E. TRUE

Psoas major inserts into the lesser trochanter

Psoas major is related posteriorly to the lumbar arteries

Ref: Last's Anatomy. McMinn 9th Edition. Churchill Livingstone.

ANSWER 29

A. TRUE   B. FALSE   C. FALSE   D. TRUE   E. FALSE

The gastroduodenal supplies the duodenum and pylorus

The left gastric artery supplies the lesser curve and fundus

Short gastric arteries arise from the splenic artery

Refs:
Last's Anatomy. McMinn. 9th Edition. Churchill Livingstone.
Anatomy for Diagnostic Imaging. Ryan & McNicholas. W B Saunders Co Ltd.

ANSWER 30

A. TRUE   B. TRUE   C. TRUE   D. TRUE   E. FALSE

The CBD joins the pancreatic duct at an angle of about 60 degrees

Refs:
Last's Anatomy. McMinn. 9th Edition. Churchill Livingstone.
Gray's Anatomy. 38th Edition. Churchill Livingstone.
Anatomy for Diagnostic Imaging. Ryan & McNicholas. W B Saunders Co Ltd.

ANSWER 31

A. FALSE   B. TRUE   C. FALSE   D. TRUE   E. TRUE

The right ureter is posterior to the third part of the duodenum

The gonadal arteries are anterior to the ureters

Ref: Last's Anatomy. McMinn. 9th Edition. Churchill Livingstone.

ANSWER 32

A. TRUE   B. FALSE   C. FALSE   D. FALSE   E. TRUE

The conus lies at L3 at birth.

The greatest diameter of the spinal cord is from side to side.

There is only one anterior spinal artery.

Refs:
Anatomy for Diagnostic Imaging. Ryan & McNicholas. W B Saunders Co Ltd.
Essential Anatomy by Lumley, Craven & Aitken. 3rd Edition. Churchill Livingstone.
Clinical Anatomy by Harold Ellis. 8th edition. Churchill Livingstone.

ANSWER 33

A. TRUE   B. FALSE   C. FALSE   D. TRUE   E. FALSE

The right pulmonary veins often unite and enter the left atrium as a single vessel.

The bronchial arteries arise from the thoracic aorta in 90% of cases.

In 80% of cases the bronchial arteries arise at T5 or T6 level.

Refs:

Anatomy for Diagnostic Imaging. Ryan & McNicholas. W B Saunders Co Ltd.
Essential Anatomy by Lumley, Craven & Aitken. 3rd Edition. Churchill Livingstone.
Clinical Anatomy by Harold Ellis. 8th edition. Churchill Livingstone.

ANSWER 34

A. FALSE   B. FALSE   C. FALSE   D. TRUE   E. TRUE

The oesophagus begins at the lower border of the cricoid cartilage.

The oesophagus is approximately is 25cm long.

The oesophagus returns to midline at level T5.

Refs:

Anatomy for Diagnostic Imaging. Ryan & McNicholas. W B Saunders Co Ltd.
Essential Anatomy by Lumley, Craven & Aitken. 3rd Edition. Churchill Livingstone.
Clinical Anatomy by Harold Ellis. 8th edition. Churchill Livingstone.

ANSWER 35

A. FALSE   B. TRUE   C. TRUE   D. TRUE   E. TRUE

This a branch of anterior cerebral artery

Refs:

Anatomy for Diagnostic Imaging. Ryan & McNicholas. W B Saunders Co Ltd.
Essential Anatomy by Lumley, Craven & Aitken. 3rd Edition. Churchill Livingstone.
Clinical Anatomy by Harold Ellis. 8th edition. Churchill Livingstone.

ANSWER 36

A. TRUE   B. TRUE   C. TRUE   D. TRUE   E. TRUE

Refs:

Anatomy for Diagnostic Imaging. Ryan & McNicholas. W B Saunders Co Ltd.
Essential Anatomy by Lumley, Craven & Aitken. 3rd Edition. Churchill Livingstone.
Clinical Anatomy by Harold Ellis. 8th edition. Churchill Livingstone.

ANSWER 37

A. TRUE   B. TRUE   C. FALSE   D. FALSE   E. FALSE

The tensor tympani tendon is attached to handle of malleus

The auditory tube opens via the anterior wall

The tegmen tympani separates the middle ear cavity from the middle cranial fossa

Refs:

Anatomy for Diagnostic Imaging. Ryan & McNicholas. W B Saunders Co Ltd.

ANSWER 38
A. TRUE   B. TRUE   C. FALSE   D. FALSE   E. TRUE

The manubriosternal joint is a secondary cartilagenous joint

The first costochrondral joint is a primary cartilagenous joint

Refs:
Anatomy for Diagnostic Imaging. Ryan & McNicholas. W B Saunders Co Ltd.
Essential Anatomy by Lumley, Craven & Aitken. 3rd Edition. Churchill Livingstone.
Clinical Anatomy by Harold Ellis. 8th edition. Churchill Livingstone.

ANSWER 39
A. TRUE   B. FALSE   C. TRUE   D. FALSE   E. TRUE

The inferior accessory fissure is seen in 8% of chest xrays

The left transverse fissure is present in 8% of the population, however it is very rarely seen on chest xrays

Refs:
Anatomy for Diagnostic Imaging. Ryan & McNicholas. W B Saunders Co Ltd.
Essential Anatomy by Lumley, Craven & Aitken. 3rd Edition. Churchill Livingstone.
Clinical Anatomy by Harold Ellis. 8th edition. Churchill Livingstone.

ANSWER 40
A. TRUE   B. TRUE   C. TRUE   D. FALSE   E. TRUE

It is supplied by the anterior division of the mandibular nerve

Refs:
Anatomy for Diagnostic Imaging. Ryan & McNicholas. W B Saunders Co Ltd.
Essential Anatomy by Lumley, Craven & Aitken. 3rd Edition. Churchill Livingstone.
Clinical Anatomy by Harold Ellis. 8th edition. Churchill Livingstone.

ANSWER 41
A. TRUE   B. TRUE   C. FALSE   D. FALSE   E. FALSE

The injection rate is 4 mls per hour. The thoracic duct should be visible in 2 hours. The maximum reduction in Tco is at 36 hours.

Ref: Whitehouse & Worthington. Techniques in Diagnostic Imaging. 3rd Edition. Blackwell Science Ltd.

ANSWER 42
A. TRUE   B. FALSE   C. TRUE   D. FALSE   E. TRUE

Uptake in bowel is intense and for this reason it may be necessary to scan the abdomen 72 hours after injection to look for intra-abdominal sepsis. Laxatives are given for two days following injection of the isotope to help clear it from the bowel.

Ref: Chapman & Nakielny. A Guide to Radiological Procedures. 3rd Edition. W B Saunders Co Ltd.

ANSWER 43

A. FALSE   B. FALSE   C. TRUE   D. FALSE   E. FALSE

8-10 MHz is more appropriate for superficial veins. The SVC is intrathoracic and therefore velocity increases during inspiration. The deep veins are more prominent with the patient standing, or sitting with the legs dependent. The popliteal vein is superficial to the artery.

Ref: Grainger & Allison. A Guide to Radiological Procedures. 3rd Edition. W B Saunders Co Ltd.

ANSWER 44

A. TRUE   B. TRUE   C. FALSE   D. TRUE   E. FALSE

Normal bladder wall thickness when empty is 0.3-0.5 cms. Renal length increases by 1 mm per week in the fetus.

Ref: Grainger & Allison. Diagnostic Radiology. 3rd Edition. Churchill Livingstone.

ANSWER 45

A. FALSE   B. TRUE   C. TRUE   D. TRUE   E. FALSE

Antegrade pyelography is performed because a retrograde pyelogram is not possible in patients with a ureteral diversion. Macroscopic haematuria is seen in 50% of cases.

Ref: Chapman & Nakielny. A Guide to Radiological Procedures. 3rd Edition. W B Saunders Co Ltd.

ANSWER 46

A. TRUE   B. TRUE   C. FALSE   D. TRUE   E. FALSE

Ref: Bell and Finlay. Basic Radiographic Positioning and Anatomy. 1st Edition. Bailliere Tindall.

ANSWER 47

A. FALSE   B. FALSE   C. TRUE   D. TRUE   E. TRUE

The right adrenal gland is more commonly visualised than the left. The adrenal cortex and medulla can be identified on ultrasound in less than 20% of patients.

Ref: Grainger & Allison. Diagnostic Radiology. 3rd Edition. Churchill Livingstone.

ANSWER 48

A. TRUE   B. FALSE   C. TRUE   D. FALSE   E. FALSE

False-negative scans occur due to filling of the gallbladder or it's assimilated appearance.

Ref: Chapman & Nakielny. A Guide to Radiological Procedures. 3rd Edition. W B Saunders Co Ltd.

ANSWER 49

A. FALSE   B. TRUE   C. FALSE   D. TRUE   E. FALSE

The left intrahepatic ducts fill preferentially in the prone position as they lie more anteriorly. The distal CBD often fails to opacify in the prone position, where contrast medium flows to the porta hepatis. 150 mg I/ml or less is required in order not to obscure small stones.

Ref: Grainger & Allison. Diagnostic Radiology. 3rd Edition. Churchill Livingston.

ANSWER 50

A. FALSE   B. TRUE   C. TRUE   D. FALSE   E. TRUE

Pancreatography is easier than retrograde cholangiography. The trickle artefact is produced during the injection of contrast into a dilated biliary tree.

Ref: Chapman & Nakielny. A Guide to Radiological Procedures. 3rd Edition. W B Saunders Co Ltd.

ANSWER 51

A. FALSE   B. TRUE   C. TRUE   D. TRUE   E. TRUE

The maximum normal jejunal calibre is 4.5 cm foe a SBE and 3.5 cms for SBM. Part E is TRUE because a thin layer of barium does not adhere as well to diseased segments.

Ref: Whitehouse & Worthington. Techniques in Diagnostic Imaging. 3rd Edition. Blackwell Science Ltd.

ANSWER 52

A. FALSE   B. FALSE   C. FALSE   D. FALSE   E. TRUE

Sections should 5mm or less. No positive rectal contrast should be used. A smooth muscle relaxant is advisable.

Ref: Grainger & Allison. Diagnostic Radiology. 3rd Edition. Churchill Livingstone.

ANSWER 53

A. FALSE   B. TRUE   C. FALSE   D. FALSE   E. TRUE

A swallow study should be performed first to localise the stricture. Femoral-visceral catheters are helpful to guide the guidewire tip through the stricture. Dilatation should be graded. Angioplasty balloons are very helpful for preliminary dilatation of tight narrow strictures.

Ref: Chapman & Nakielny. A Guide to Radiological Procedures. 3rd Edition. 1993. W B Saunders Co Ltd.

ANSWER 54

A. TRUE   B. FALSE   C. TRUE   D. FALSE   E. FALSE

The sidearms are for flushing catheters with saline, heparin or for drug infusion. The main indication is to allow muultiole catheter changes. Very helpful to do check angiograms during thrombolysis studies. Protects vessel from damage by the balloon.

Ref: Chapman & Nakielny. A Guide to Radiological Procedures. 3rd Edition. W B Saunders Co Ltd.

ANSWER 55
A. FALSE   B. TRUE   C. FALSE   D. TRUE   E. TRUE

IVC filters come with their own sheath. A venogram is required to confirm that there is no thrombus at the site of puncture, check that there is no distal thrombus, and measures the size of the IVC. If it is over 2.5 - 3 cms, this is a contraindication for insertion of standard caval filters. There are specific temporary caval filters which can be left in for longer than 12 -14 days. A birds nest filter is the only caval filter at present which can be inserted into a megacava (> 3 cm).

Ref: Chapman & Nakielny. A Guide to Radiological Procedures. 3rd Edition. W B Saunders Co Ltd.

ANSWER 56
A. TRUE   B. TRUE   C. FALSE   D. FALSE   E. FALSE

Sagittal sequences are poor at looking at TFCC. Axial images are ususally T1 or T2* or STIR sequences.

Ref: MRI in Orthopaedics and Sports Medicine. Stoller. Lippincott Raven.

ANSWER 57
A. FALSE   B. FALSE   C. TRUE   D. TRUE   E. FALSE

Time activity curver are created from the the arterial phase. The blood pool phase is a single image at 5 minutes lasting 3 minutes. Reconstruction is only performed if an abnormality is seen. A dynamic image can be obtained in the first 20-30 minutes which will give an indication of renal function. No significant complications are known.

Ref: Chapman & Nakielny. A Guide to Radiological Procedures. 3rd Edition. W B Saunders Co Ltd.

ANSWER 58
A. TRUE   B. TRUE   C. FALSE   D. TRUE   E. FALSE

The centering point for an AP view of the ankle is the medial malleolus and for the AP view of the foot is the middle cunieform.

Ref: Bell & Finlay. Basic Radiographic Positioning & Anatomy. 1st Edition. Bailliere Tindall.

ANSWER 59
A. FALSE   B. TRUE   C. FALSE   D. TRUE   E. FALSE

LAO or RPO views are performed of the left lung, and a TRUE lateral of the right. The right lung should be imaged before the left so that a lateral can be taken without superimposition of the left lung. Nowadays spot views should be taken as water soluble contrast is less viscous.

Ref: Chapman & Nakielny. A Guide to Radiological Procedures. 3rd Edition. W B Saunders Co Ltd.

ANSWER 60
A. TRUE   B. TRUE   C. TRUE   D. TRUE   E. TRUE

Ref: Chapman & Nakielny. A Guide to Radiological Procedures. 3rd Edition. W B Saunders Co Ltd.

Exam 5

QUESTION 1

Regarding x-ray film

A. Silver halide is sensitive in the blue part of the visible spectrum
B. The spectral sensitivity of silver halide can be altered by adding certain light absorbing dyes to the emulsions
C. A latent image is only produced after the film has been both exposed and developed
D. The speed of an emulsion is predominantly dependent on the grain size distribution
E. In the film emulsion there is an excess of silver bromide compared to silver iodide

QUESTION 2

Regarding the Geiger-Muller (GM) tube

A. Halogen gas is added to the inert gas
B. The gas is maintained at low pressure
C. The tube requires to be operated at voltages in the plateau region
D. The potential difference across the tube ranges from 200-400 volts to 900-1500 volts
E. The GM counter is able to distinguish between different types of radiation

QUESTION 3

Regarding x-ray generating apparatus

A. The kVp meter is located in the control panel
B. The mA meter is located in the control panel
C. The kVp meter is incorporated into the high voltage circuit of the x-ray generator
D. The mA meter is incorporated into the high voltage circuit of the x-ray generator
E. The high voltage circuit of an x-ray generator consists of a single transformer

QUESTION 4

Regarding attenuation of an x-ray beam

A. This occurs solely by absorption of photons
B. In the attenuation of monochromatic radiation, both the number of photons in the beam and the energy of the photons are reduced
C. Attenuation of monochromatic radiation is exponential
D. Attenuation of polychromatic radiation is exponential
E. Attenuation of polychromatic radiation results in beam hardening

QUESTION 5
Regarding xeroradiography

A. In this process the detecting medium used is the charged surface of an amorphous selenium photoconducting plate
B. The latent electrostatic image is developed in the same way as photographic x-ray film
C. Following use, the selenium plates are stored in an uncharged state prior to re-use
D. Xeroradiography can produce either "positive" or "negative" images
E. A xeroradiographic process has a very narrow exposure latitude when compared to conventional film screen systems

QUESTION 6
Regarding grids used in diagnostic radiography

A. A grid with a lower grid ratio is more efficient at removing scatter radiation compared to a high ratio grid
B. A high ratio grid has a higher bucky factor
C. Primary transmission refers to the amount of primary radiation absorbed by the grid
D. Primary transmission of a grid is inversely proportionate to grid ratio
E. There is always some loss of the transmission in primary radiation caused by a grid

QUESTION 7
Regarding the structure of an atom

A. The number of electrons in the M electron shell is 8
B. The binding energy of an M shell electron is greater than that of an L shell electron
C. An isotope is a substance with the same number of protons but different number of neutrons
D. Isotopes have identical physical properties but different chemical properties
E. The number of neutrons in an atom, N, is equal to A-Z

QUESTION 8
Interactions of x-rays with matter

A. The second half value layer (HVL) of a material is usually less than the first HVL
B. The HVL of a typical diagnostic x-ray beam is 30cm in tissue
C. As an x-ray beam penetrates a material it becomes progressively more heterogeneous
D. The photoelectric effect results from an interaction with a free electron
E. Compton scattering is independent of electron density

QUESTION 9
Tube rating

A. Increases as the effective "focal spot" size increases
B. Increases as the kV increases
C. Is greater for a high speed anode assembly compared to a routine rotating assembly
D. In continuous operation fluoroscopy, rating is partly dependent on the focal spot size
E. Is greater for a 3 phase generator compared to a single phase generator

QUESTION 10

The following regarding film processing are true

A. The steps involved in film processing are fixation, washing, developing, washing and finally drying
B. The developer is usually an alkaline solution of a reducing agent
C. Following "developing" the film is opaque
D. Film is 'fixed' with an acid solution of thiosulphate
E. Incomplete fixation usually leaves the film brown/yellow

QUESTION 11

Macroradiography

A. To obtain a magnified image, the focus-object distance is decreased relative to the object film distance which is increased
B. A very small focal spot must be used
C. A grid is routinely used
D. Usually results in reduced patient dose
E. Quantum mottle is not increased

QUESTION 12

Regarding intensifying screens

A. X-ray absorption in an intensifying screen is about 30% for Tungstate and 60% for rare earth screens
B. Screen efficiency for screens is about 50%
C. Screen conversion efficiency is about 20% for Tungstate and 50% for rare earth screens
D. Increasing the conversion efficiency of a screen reduces quantum mottle
E. Increasing screen thickness increases quantum mottle

QUESTION 13

Television systems used in image intensification

A. The photoconducting material in the videcon tube is lead monoxide
B. The photoconducting material used in the plumbicon tube is lead monoxide
C. The image intensifier exhibits a longer "lag" period than the TV camera tube
D. In cine-radiography a frame rate of greater than 16 per second is sufficient to prevent jerky motion
E. The dose to the patient when using 70/100mm photospot film, is 3-5 times smaller than with full size (puck) film

QUESTION 14

Regarding detectors used in computed tomography (CT)

A. Calcium fluoride may be used as the scintillation crystals in a CT detector
B. Bismuth germanate may be used as the scintillation crystals in a CT detector
C. Ionization chambers are more sensitive than scintillation detectors
D. Scintillation detectors are more stable to voltage fluctuation compared to ionization chambers
E. Ionization chambers are well suited to the fourth generation type of CT scanners

QUESTION 15

Regarding radionuclides and their effective doses

A. ^{99m}T- macroaggregates of albumin: effective dose (ED) - 5 mSv
B. ^{67}Galium: ED - 18 mSv
C. ^{99m}Tc MAG3: ED - 1 mSv
D. ^{81m}Kr gas: ED - 1 mSv
E. ^{99m}Tc phosphonates: ED - 1 mSv

QUESTION 16

The following entrance doses are appropriate for the following radiographs

A. AP lumbar spine x-ray: 10 mGy
B. AP abdominal x-ray: 5mGy
C. AP pelvic x-ray: 5 mGy
D. PA chest x-ray: 0.3 mGy
E. PA skull x-ray: 5 mGy

QUESTION 17

The following statements are true

A. Protons in fat have a relatively short T1
B. T2 is the time for the MR signal to fall to 63% of its maximum value
C. A typical T2 relaxation time for CSF is 150 ms
D. A typical T1 relaxation time for CSF is 150 ms
E. Compact bone has a very long T2

QUESTION 18

Regarding the inversion recovery (IR) sequence in MRI

A. An initial 90 degree radio frequency pulse is followed, after a time TI, by a 180 degree pulse
B. Generally speaking, the signal received in an IR sequence is T2 weighted
C. The longer the T1 of a tissue, the greater the MR signal produced
D. The longer the TI the greater the MRI signal produced
E. TI is used as a T1 contrast control

QUESTION 19
Spectroscopic imaging of phosphorus- 31 (^{31}P)

A. ^{31}P has a larger gyromagnetic ratio than hydrogen at 1T
B. Necessitates the use of a super conducting magnet
C. Allows the study of ^{31}P metabolism in vivo
D. Requires a uniform field of at least 10 parts per million
E. Image resolution is much worse than in conventional MRI

QUESTION 20
Persons may receive higher radiation doses in the following types of work

A. Cardiac catheterisation
B. Interventional radiology
C. Radiopharmaceutical preparation
D. Nursing a patient undergoing brachytherapy
E. Preparation and insertion of radioactive implants

QUESTION 21
Regarding the pituitary gland

A. Its stalk is composed of nerve fibres whose cell bodies are in the third ventricle
B. The anterior lobe is five times larger than the posterior lobe
C. The posterior lobe develops from rathke's pouch
D. Its superior relations are diaphragm sella and optic chiasm
E. The inter-cavernous sinus does not surround the pituitary gland superiorly

QUESTION 22
Regarding the bones of the leg

A. The attachment of the patellar ligament is part of the tibial epiphysis
B. The tibial shaft is triangular in cross-section
C. In children the fibula is proportionally thinner than in adults
D. The malleolar fossa of the fibula is seen on the antero-medial aspect of the lateral malleolus
E. The tibia is grooved posteriorly by the tibialis posterior tendon

QUESTION 23
The following are supplied by the femoral nerve

A. Gracilis
B. Iliacus
C. Vastus lateralis
D. Gluteus minimus
E. Tensor fascia lata

QUESTION 24

Regarding ossification times

A. The radial head is fused at 17 years
B. The distal ulnar epiphysis is present at birth
C. None of the carpal bones are ossified at birth
D. The centre for the trochlea appears at 10 years
E. The scaphoid is the first carpal bone to ossify

QUESTION 25

The following are true of upper limb veins

A. The cephalic vein runs on the lateral side of the forearm
B. The basilic vein pierces the clavipectoral fascia to join the axillary vein
C. The median cubital vein connects the cephalic vein to deep brachial veins
D. There are usually two venae comitantes following the course of the subclavian artery
E. The median forearm vein runs along the dorsum of the forearm

QUESTION 26

The rectum

A. Is about 20 cm long
B. Becomes continuous with the sigmoid colon at the level of the third sacral segment
C. Is not covered with peritoneum
D. Has four rectal valves (of Houston)
E. Derives its blood supply from superior, middle and inferior rectal arteries

QUESTION 27

The following statements are true regarding the sigmoid colon

A. It has its own mesentery
B. Lymphatic drainage is to para-aortic nodes
C. It usually measures less than 45 cm
D. There is a change in mucosal pattern between rectum and sigmoid colon
E. The limbs of the sigmoid mesocolon diverge at the bifurcation of the right common iliac artery

QUESTION 28

The appendix

A. Commonly opens into the posteromedial wall of the caecum
B. Is supplied by a branch of the inferior mesenteric artery
C. Has its own mesentery
D. Commonly measures less than 3 cm in length
E. Has a collateral arterial supply

QUESTION 29

On a CT scan at the level of L1

A. The body of the pancreas lies on the splenic vein
B. The inferior vena cava is seen closely related to the caudate lobe of the liver
C. The superior mesenteric artery leaves the aorta
D. The right adrenal gland is usually visible
E. Segment II of the liver is usually visible

QUESTION 30

The left renal vein lies posterior to

A. Abdominal aorta
B. Body of pancreas
C. Third part of duodenum
D. Superior mesenteric artery
E. Left renal artery

QUESTION 31

Anterior relations of the right kidney include

A. Quadrate lobe of liver
B. Duodenum
C. Ascending colon
D. Ascending branch of right colic artery
E. Segment II of the liver

QUESTION 32

The following statements are true

A. The arachnoid mater is thickened laterally between the nerve roots as the denticulate ligament
B. The dural or thecal sac extends up to the S2 vertebral level
C. The posterior spinal arteries supplies two thirds of the cross sectional area of the spinal cord
D. The posterior spinal arteries arise more commonly from the posterior inferior cerebellar branches rather than vertebral arteries
E. The artery radicularis magna or the artery of Adamkiewicz commonly arises from the left side

QUESTION 33

The following statements are true

A. The left atrium is the most posterior chamber in the heart
B. The tricuspid and mitral valves are roughly vertically orientated
C. The normal pericardial sac contains 50 mls of serous fluid
D. The visceral layer of the pericardium is also known as the epicardium
E. The pericardium extends on to the SVC up to azygous vein insertion

QUESTION 34

The following are true

A. The upper one third of oesophagus is supplied by the inferior thyroid artery
B. The lower one third of oesophagus is supplied by the descending aorta
C. The oesophagus has striated muscle in its upper one third
D. The venous drainage of middle one third of oesophagus is to the azygous system
E. The venous drainage of lower one third of oesophagus is to the left gastric vein

QUESTION 35

The following statements are true

A. The anterior wall of third ventricle is partly formed by lamina terminalis
B. The massa intermedia is a grey matter tract
C. The habenular commissure is anterior to the pineal gland
D. The foramen of magendie connect lateral and third ventricles
E. The third ventricle is a cavity of mesencephalon

QUESTION 36

Regarding the cranial venous sinuses

A. The superior sagittal sinus usually joins the left transverse sinus
B. The inferior sagittal sinus joins the right transverse sinus
C. The straight sinus usually joins the left transverse sinus
D. The two transverse sinuses often communicate at the internal occipital protuberance
E. The cavernous sinus is traversed by the internal carotid artery

QUESTION 37

Regarding the inner ear

A. The bony labyrinth comprises of cochlea, vestibule and the semicircular canals
B. The cochlea is situated posterior to the vestibule
C. The lateral wall of vestibule opens into the middle ear at the round and oval window
D. There are six openings into the vestibule via the three semicircular canals
E. The saccule lies in the cochlea and the utricle lies in the vestibule

QUESTION 38

The following statements are true

A. The internal thoracic artery ends at the sixth intercostal space
B. At the origin of internal thoracic artery it is crossed by the phrenic nerve
C. The internal thoracic artery divides into musculophrenic and subcostal arteries
D. There are two anterior and one posterior intercostal vein for each intercostal space
E. The internal thoracic artery gives anterior intercostal artery to upper six spaces

QUESTION 39
The following statements are true

A. The minor fissure is 1cm below the hilar point
B. The normal hilar angle at the hilar point is 120 degrees
C. The cricopharyngeal impression is seen in 5% of normal studies
D. The right paraspinal line is thicker than the left side
E. The pulmonary veins in the first intercostal space are up to 3mm in size

QUESTION 40
Regarding the nasal cavity

A. The vomer forms the anterosuperior part of the nasal septum
B. The middle and inferior conchae are part of the ethmoid bone
C. The floor of the nasal cavity is at a lower level than the floor of the maxillary sinus
D. The perpendicular plate of the palatine bone contributes to the septum
E. The sphenoidal sinus is in its roof

QUESTION 41
Regarding venography

A. AP and oblique views of the saphenofemoral junction are required during peripheral varicography
B. A rapid injection of 30 mls into a medial anterior cubital fossa vein will adequately opacify the superior venacava
C. Clot dislodgement commonly causes PE during venography
D. MRI can be used to age venous thrombus
E. Bilateral femoral vein puncture is required to image the inferior venacava

QUESTION 42
Regarding gestational dating with ultrasound

A. Head circumference measurements are less accurate than the biparietal diameter
B. Biparietal diameter is most reliable in the third trimester
C. Crown rump length is most reliable in the first trimester
D. The yolk sac is reliably detected by transvaginal ultrasound at four weeks gestation
E. The heart beat is not reliably detected before 6.5 weeks on transabdominal ultrasound

QUESTION 43
Mag-3 renograms

A. Can be used to demonstrate renal scarring following infection
B. Allows estimation of the glomerular filtration rate
C. Mag-3 is 80% passively filtered at the glomerulus
D. A bolus of intravenous frusemide at 10 minutes allows differentiation between a dilated non-obstructed system and an obstructed one
E. Images are required at 20-30 minutes following isotope injection

QUESTION 44

Regarding Discography

A. Prophylactic antibiotics are indicated
B. The patient should be well sedated
C. Discography of a normal disc is painless
D. 2 mls non-ionic contrast media are injected into the nucleus pulposus
E. Retroperitoneal haemorrhage is a recognised complication

QUESTION 45

The following are true regarding a Towne's view of the skull (30 degrees fronto-occipital)

A. The radiographic baseline is at 90 degrees to the cassette
B. Tube angulation is in the cranial direction
C. The dorsum sellae is projected through the foramen magnum
D. The zygomatic arches are not visible
E. The coronal suture is not visible

QUESTION 46

Whem imaging the adrenal glands

A. Ultrasound is the modality of choice in children
B. The spacial resolution of MRI is greater than CT
C. ^{75}Se-cholesterol is predominantly taken up by the adrenal medulla
D. ^{123}I-MIBG is predominantly taken up by the adrenal cortex
E. ^{123}I-MIBG uptake in the lungs is normal

QUESTION 47

The following statements are true

A. Coopers ligament are invisible on ultrasound of the breast
B. During Doppler venography, the valsalva manouvre does not transmit below the knee
C. The paramedial lobe of the thyroid arises from the superior aspect of the isthmus
D. An intervening loop of bowel is an absolute contraindication to fine needle aspiration
E. The upper limit for normal for AP diameter of the aorta in a 60 year old is 2.5 cm

QUESTION 48

Regarding liver scintigraphy

A. Planar imaging can detect lesions 2 cm in size
B. SPECT can detect lesions 5 mm in size
C. The normal liver is visualised before the spleen
D. Is indicated in the diagnosis of renal transplant rejection
E. Colloid shift is the abnormal redistribution of isotope into the biliary tree

QUESTION 49

Regarding endoscopic retrograde cholangiopancreatography

A. A prolonged prothombin time is a contraindication
B. Duodenal hypotension aids papilla cannulation
C. The procedure is more prone to technical failure than percutaneous transhepatic cholangiography
D. The pancreatic tree should be visualised before the biliary tree
E. Aspiration pneumonitis is a complication

QUESTION 50

The following are absolute contraindications

A. Barium swallow - oesophageal leak into pleura
B. Barium swallow - aspiration
C. Gastrograffin - aspiration
D. Gastromiro - aspiration
E. Barium swallow - peritoneal leak

QUESTION 51

Barium Swallow - Double contrast

A. Views of the stomach are mandatory
B. Views of the upper oesophagus are mandatory
C. Turn patient to left side to look for reflux
D. AP views mandatory
E. Lateral view is mandatory

QUESTION 52

Properties of Barium enema suspension are

A. Particle size is large approximately 4.5 micrometers
B. Particles are coated with agents
C. Slow flow is preferable
D. The suspension should provide plastic coating characteristics
E. Should contain antifoaming agents

QUESTION 53

Ultrasound of oesophagus

A. A 5 MHz transducer is used
B. A 90 degree rotatory transducer is required
C. Stomach filled with warm tap water
D. Rotatory transducer provides excellent transverse views of oesophagus
E. Should be monitored with pulse oximeter

QUESTION 54

The angiographic unit must have a

A. High speed rotating cathode
B. Focal spot of 0.1 - 0.2 mm sq
C. Floating table top
D. Biplane unit
E. Tilting table top

QUESTION 55

Patient preparation for angiography includes

A. Premedication
B. Written consent
C. Blood glucose assessment
D. ECG monitoring
E. Nil by mouth for 4 hours

QUESTION 56

Routine MRI of ankle sequences include

A. Coronal T1
B. Coronal STIR
C. Sagittal GE
D. Axial T1
E. Coronal T2

QUESTION 57

Regarding hip Arthrography

A. 6-10 mls of contrast is introduced in an adult
B. 6-10 mls air is introduced in an adult
C. Lateral approach routine
D. Active movement
E. Frogs view for children helpful

QUESTION 58

The half-life of the following radioisotopes are appropriate

A. ^{81m}Krypton - 30 sec
B. ^{133}Xenon - 5.25 days
C. ^{127}Xenon - 2 weeks
D. ^{113m}Indium - 30 seconds
E. ^{111m}Indium - 2.8 days

QUESTION 59
CT Pulmonary Angiogram

A. Requires 70 mls non-ionic contrast media
B. A pump injection of 2 mls per second is used
C. The scan should start at the level of the arch of the aorta
D. High resolution algorithm is required
E. A HRCT scan should be performed first

QUESTION 60
The following centering points are correct

A. Axial elbow - 5cm distal to the olecranon
B. AP shoulder - head of humerus
C. Lateral toes - midshaft of 1st metatarsal
D. Lateral foot - base of fifth metatarsal
E. Lateral view of the calcaneus - middle of calcaneus

Exam 5: Answers

ANSWER 1
A. TRUE   B. TRUE   C. FALSE   D. FALSE   E. TRUE

The latent image is formed following an exposure and before development

The speed of an emulsion is largely dependent on the average size of the grains rather than the grain size distribution. The greater the average grain size the greater the speed of the emulsion.

Film emulsion contains approx. 90% silver bromide and 10% of silver iodide

Ref: Curry & Thomas. Christensen's Physics of Diagnostic Radiology. 4th Edition. Williams & Wilkins (Europe) Ltd.

ANSWER 2
A. TRUE   B. TRUE   C. TRUE   D. TRUE   E. FALSE

The GM counter is able to detect any ionising radiation but does not distinguish between different types, nor can it distinguish between energies of the same radiation

Ref: Curry & Thomas. Christensen's Physics of Diagnostic Radiology. 4th Edition. Williams & Wilkins (Europe) Ltd.

ANSWER 3
A. TRUE   B. TRUE   C. TRUE   D. TRUE   E. FALSE

Whilst both the kVp meter and mA meter are located in the control panel, their connections are in the high voltage circuit. The high voltage circuit of an x-ray generator consists of two transformers, an autotransformer and a step-up transformer. The kVp meter is placed in the circuit between the autotransformer and the step-up transformer, and therefore only needs a minimum of insulation when placed in the control panel. However for the mA meter to provide accurate mA recordings, the connections for the mA meter need to be in the secondary coil of the transformer. Hence the connections need to be grounded

Ref: Armstrong. Lecture Notes on the Physics of Radiology. 1st Edition. 1990. Clinical Press Ltd.

ANSWER 4
A. FALSE   B. FALSE   C. TRUE   D. FALSE   E. TRUE

Attenuation occurs either by absorption of photons, or scattering of photons from the beam

Attenutaion of monochromatic radiation does not change the quality of the radiation. However, the number of the photons in the beam is reduced

Attenuation of polychromatic radiation is not exponential, i.e. the number of photons remaining in the beam does not decrease by the same percentage with each increment of absorber. When the percentage of transmission is plotted on semi-log paper it is curved (as opposed to with monochromatic radiation which is a straight line)

Ref: Armstrong: Lecture Notes on the Physics of Radiology. 1st Edition 1990. Clinical Press Ltd.

ANSWER 5

A. TRUE   B. FALSE   C. TRUE   D. TRUE   E. FALSE

The electrostatic image is developed by exposing the surface of the plate to a fine charged powder called "toner" which is attracted to the plate surface in proportion to the intensity of the remaining charge. As the toner particles have both positive and negative charges it is possible to attract either of these selectively to the surface of the plate to produce either a positive or negative image

The process has very broad exposure latitudes. The resolution is less sensitive to exposure and hence a single exposure can produce good image resolution in both thick and thin areas of a structure i.e. the breast

Ref: Armstrong. Lecture Notes on the Physics of Radiology. 1st Edition. 1990. Clinical Press Ltd.

ANSWER 6

A. FALSE   B. TRUE   C. TRUE   D. TRUE   E. TRUE

High ratio grids are more efficient at removing scattered radiation

As the bucky factor is the ratio of incident radiation to transmitted radiation, high ratio grids also have a larger bucky factor. Grid ratio refers to how efficient a grid is at removing secondary (scattered) radiation

Whilst it is desirable for a grid to only prevent the passage of secondary scattered radiation, there is always some absorption of primary radiation. Hence when using a grid, exposure factors need to be increased

Ref: Armstrong. Lecture Notes on the Physics of Radiology. 1st Edition. Clinical Press Ltd.

ANSWER 7

A. FALSE   B. FALSE   C. TRUE   D. FALSE   E. TRUE

The number of electrons in the M shell is 18

K > L > M. Energy (E):K = 70, E:L = 11, E:M = 2 keV

Isotopes have identical chemical properties

Where A is the mass number and Z is the atomic number

Ref: Farr & Allisy-Roberts. Physics for Medical Imaging. 1st Edition. W B Saunders Co Ltd.

ANSWER 8

A. FALSE   B. FALSE   C. FALSE   D. FALSE   E. FALSE

With each HVL, the average energy of the photons increases - the beam becomes "harder" or more penetrating. The second HVL is larger than the first HVL

The HVL of a typical diagnostic beam is 30mm

As an x-ray beam penetrates a material it becomes progressively more homogenous secondary to beam hardening

The photoelectric effect results from interactions with "bound" inner shell electrons

The probability that the Compton process will occur is proportional to the physical density and in particular electron density, and is inversely proportional to the incident photon energy. It is independent of Z

Ref: Farr & Allisy-Roberts. Physics for Medical Imaging. 1st Edition. W B Saunders Co Ltd.

ANSWER 9

A. TRUE   B. FALSE   C. TRUE   D. FALSE   E. TRUE

The rating decreases as the kV is increased

At higher speeds, heat is more evenly spread along the focal track resulting in greater rating

In continuous fluoroscopy, the rating depends only on the rate of cooling of the tube and not upon focal spot size or type of generator used

Tube rating is about 35% greater with 3 phase generators compared to single phase generators

Ref: Farr & Allisy-Roberts. Physics for Medical Imaging. 1st Edition. W B Saunders Co Ltd.

ANSWER 10

A. FALSE   B. TRUE   C. TRUE   D. TRUE   E. FALSE

The steps in processing are developer, washing, fixing, washing and finally drying

Developer:- for example, sodium hydroxide and sodium carbonate, electron donors to convert the latent image into metallic silver

The solution of thiosulphate is also known as "hypo"

Incomplete fixation leaves the film "milky". Incomplete washing leaves the film brown/yellow

Ref: Farr & Allisy-Roberts. Physics for Medical Imaging. 1st Edition. W B Saunders Co Ltd.

ANSWER 11

A. TRUE   B. TRUE   C. FALSE   D. FALSE   E. TRUE

A very small focal spot decreases geometric unsharpness

The air gap technique is usually employed

There is increased patient dose due to the increased exposure factors required

Quantum mottle is not increased since the same number of x-ray photons are absorbed in the screen for the same degree of film blackening

Ref: Farr & Allisy-Roberts. Physics for Medical Imaging. 1st Edition. W B Saunders Co Ltd.

ANSWER 12

A. TRUE   B. TRUE   C. FALSE   D. FALSE   E. FALSE

Screen efficiency is the proportion of light produced in a screen that reaches the film

Screen conversion efficiency is 5% for Tungstate screens and 20% for rare earth screens

When using a thicker screen, the same number of x-ray photons are absorbed in the screen for the same film density. Hence there is no change in noise although resolution is reduced. When the conversion or screen efficiency is increased, a reduced number of x-ray photons are required to be absorbed for the same film density. Hence exposure required and patient dose are reduced, but noise is increased. Increasing screen efficiency reduces resolution but increasing conversion efficiency does not affect resolution.

Thus increasing conversion efficiency increases quantum noise but increasing screen thickness does not affect noise; however both increase the speed of a screen and reduce patient dose.

Ref: Farr & Allisy-Roberts. Physics for Medical Imaging. 1st Edition. W B Saunders Co Ltd.

ANSWER 13

A. FALSE   B. TRUE   C. FALSE   D. TRUE   E. TRUE

The vidicon tube uses antimony trisulphide as the photoconducting material

The image intensifier has a "lag" period of about 1ms. The camera tube may have a "lag" of several hundred ms

50 frames per second is necessary to eliminate flicker altogether

Ref: Farr & Allisy-Roberts. Physics for Medical Imaging. 1st Edition. W B Saunders Co Ltd.

ANSWER 14

A. TRUE   B. TRUE   C. FALSE   D. FALSE   E. FALSE

NaI, CsI, CdW may also be used as scintillation crystals in a CT detector

Scintillation detectors are more sensitive than ionization chambers

Ionization chambers are more stable to voltage fluctuation compared to scintillation detectors

Ionization chambers are more suitable for third generation scanners. Solid state detectors are more appropriate for fourth generation scanners

Ref: Farr & Allisy-Roberts. Physics for Medical Imaging. 1st Edition. W B Saunders Co Ltd.

ANSWER 15

A. FALSE   B. TRUE   C. TRUE   D. FALSE   E. FALSE

^{99m}Tc MAA: ED - 1 mSv

^{81m}Kr: ED - 0.1 mSv

^{99m}Tc phosphonates: ED - 5 mSv

Ref: Farr & Allisy-Roberts. Physics for Medical Imaging. 1st Edition. W B Saunders Co Ltd.

ANSWER 16

A. TRUE   B. FALSE   C. FALSE   D. TRUE   E. TRUE

AP abdomen: 10 mGy

AP pelvis: 10 mGy

Ref: Farr & Allisy-Roberts. Physics for Medical Imaging. 1st Edition. W B Saunders Co Ltd.

ANSWER 17
A. TRUE   B. FALSE   C. TRUE   D. FALSE   E. FALSE

T2 is the time for the MR signal to fall to 37% of its maximum value

T1 relaxation for CSF: - 2,000 ms

Compact bone, tendons, teeth and metallic clips all have a very short T2 and do not produce a lasting signal

Ref: Farr & Allisy-Roberts. Physics for Medical Imaging. 1st Edition. W B Saunders Co Ltd.

ANSWER 18
A. FALSE   B. FALSE   C. FALSE   D. TRUE   E. TRUE

There is an initial 180 degree pulse followed by a 90 degree pulse after TI

These sequences are generally T1 weighted

Greater MR signal is produced with tissues which have a short T1

Ref: Farr & Allisy-Roberts. Physics for Medical Imaging. 1st Edition. W B Saunders Co Ltd.

ANSWER 19
A. FALSE   B. TRUE   C. TRUE   D. FALSE   E. TRUE

Gyromagnetic ratio: ^{31}P = 17.2 MHz, H: 42.6 MHz

High field strengths (2T or more) are required, hence the need for superconducting magnets

The uniformity of the field should be better than 1 part per million

To reduce imaging time, large pixels in a coarse matrix (1cm pixels) must be used and consequently image resolution is much worse than in conventional MRI

Ref: Farr & Allisy-Roberts. Physics for Medical Imaging. 1st Edition. W B Saunders Co Ltd.

ANSWER 20
A. TRUE   B. TRUE   C. TRUE   D. TRUE   E. TRUE

It is unlikely that many persons in a hospital will need to be designated as classified persons on the basis of likely exposure. However, in the types of work listed, persons may receive higher doses.

Ref: Regulation 9 AC1/64. The Ionising Radiations Regulations 1988 (IRR 88).

ANSWER 21
A. TRUE   B. TRUE   C. FALSE   D. TRUE   E. TRUE

It is the anterior lobe that develops from rathke's pouch which is located in the roof of the primitive mouth.

Refs:
Anatomy for Diagnostic Imaging. Ryan & McNicholas. W B Saunders Co Ltd.
Essential Anatomy by Lumley, Craven & Aitken. 3rd Edition, Churchill Livingstone.
Clinical Anatomy by Harold Ellis. 8th Edition. Churchill Livingstone.

ANSWER 22

A. TRUE   B. TRUE   C. FALSE   D. FALSE   E. TRUE

The fibula is proportionally thicker in children

The malleolar fossa is on the postero-medial aspect of the medial malleolus

Refs:
Last's Anatomy. McMinn. 9th Edition. Churchill Livingstone.
Gray's Anatomy. 38th Edition. Churchill Livingstone.

ANSWER 23

A. FALSE   B. TRUE   C. TRUE   D. FALSE   E. FALSE

Gracilis is supplied by the obturator nerve

Gluteus minimus is supplied by the superior gluteal nerve

Tensor fascia lata is supplied by the superior gluteal nerve

Ref: Last's Anatomy. McMinn. 9th Edition. Churchill Livingstone.

ANSWER 24

A. TRUE   B. FALSE   C. TRUE   D. TRUE   E. FALSE

The dital ulnar epiphysis appears at about 5-6 years

The capitate is first carpal bone to ossify

Ref: Last's Anatomy. McMinn 9th Edition. Churchill Livingstone.

ANSWER 25

A. TRUE   B. FALSE   C. FALSE   D. FALSE   E. FALSE

The cephalic vein pierces the clavipectoral fascia to join the axillary vein

The median cubital vein connects the cephalic to the basilic vein

Usually a single subclavian vein follows the course of the subclavian artery

The median forearm vein runs along the ventral aspect of the forearm

Refs:
Last's Anatomy. McMinn. 9th Edition. Churchill Livingstone.
Anatomy for Diagnostic Imaging. Ryan & McNicholas. W B Saunders Co Ltd.

ANSWER 26

A. FALSE   B. TRUE   C. FALSE   D. FALSE   E. TRUE

The rectum is about 12 cm long

The upper third of the rectum is covered with peritoneum anteriorly and laterally

There are three rectal valves

Ref: Last's Anatomy. McMinn. 9th Edition. Churchill Livingstone

ANSWER 27

A. TRUE   B. FALSE   C. TRUE   D. FALSE   E. FALSE

Lymphatic drainage is to inferior mesenteric nodes

There is no change in mucosal pattern between the rectum and sigmoid

The limbs diverge at the bifurcation of the left common iliac artery

Refs:
Last's Anatomy. McMinn. 9th Edition. Churchill Livingstone.
Anatomy for Diagnostic Imaging. Ryan & McNicholas. W B Saunders Co Ltd.

ANSWER 28

A. TRUE   B. FALSE   C. TRUE   D. FALSE   E. FALSE

The appendix is supplied by the iliocolic artery from the superior mesenteric artery

The appendix normally measures 6-9 cm in length

The appendicular artery is an end artery

Refs:
Last's Anatomy. McMinn. 9th Edition. Churchill Livingstone.
Gray's Anatomy. 38th Edition. Churchill Livingstone.

ANSWER 29

A. TRUE   B. FALSE   C. TRUE   D. FALSE   E. FALSE

The inferior vena cava is free of the liver at L1

The right adrenal gland lies higher around T11

Segment II of the liver is seen between T10 and T11

Refs:
Last's Anatomy. McMinn. 9th Edition. Churchill Livingstone.
Anatomy for Diagnostic Imaging. Ryan & McNicholas. W B Saunders Co Ltd.
Imaging Atlas of Human Anatomy. Weir & Abrahams. 2nd Edition. Mosby.

ANSWER 30

A. FALSE   B. TRUE   C. FALSE   D. TRUE   E. FALSE

The renal vein is anterior to the abdominal aorta

The renal vein is superior to the third part of the duodenum

The renal vein is anterior to the left renal artery

Refs:
Last's Anatomy. McMinn. 9th Edition. Churchill Livingstone.
Gray's Anatomy. 38th Edition. Churchill Livingstone.

ANSWER 31
A. FALSE B. TRUE C. TRUE D. TRUE E. FALSE

The quadrate lobe lies more medial in relation to the right kidney

Segment II is part of the left lobe of the liver

Refs:
Last's Anatomy. McMinn. 9th Edition. Churchill Livingstone.
Gray's Anatomy. 38th Edition. Churchill Livingstone.
Anatomy for Diagnostic Imaging. Ryan & McNicholas. W B Saunders Co Ltd.

ANSWER 32
A. FALSE B. TRUE C. FALSE D. TRUE E. TRUE

The denticulate ligament arises from pia mater.

Two thirds of the cross sectional area of the spinal cord is supplied by the single anterior spinal artery

Refs:
Anatomy for Diagnostic Imaging. Ryan & McNicholas. W B Saunders Co Ltd.
Essential Anatomy by Lumley,Craven & Aitken. 3rd Edition,Churchill Livingstone.
Clinical Anatomy by Harold Ellis. 8th Edition. Churchill Livingstone.

ANSWER 33
A. TRUE B. TRUE C. FALSE D. TRUE E. TRUE

The pericardial sac normally contains 20-25 mls only.

Refs:
Anatomy for Diagnostic Imaging. Ryan & McNicholas. W B Saunders Co Ltd.
Essential Anatomy by Lumley,Craven & Aitken. 3rd Edition,Churchill Livingstone.
Clinical Anatomy by Harold Ellis. 8th Edition. Churchill Livingstone.

ANSWER 34
A. TRUE B. FALSE C. TRUE D. TRUE E. TRUE

Lower one third is supplied by left gastric artery.

Refs:
Anatomy for Diagnostic Imaging. Ryan & McNicholas. W B Saunders Co Ltd.
Essential Anatomy by Lumley,Craven & Aitken. 3rd Edition,Churchill Livingstone.
Clinical Anatomy by Harold Ellis. 8th Edition. Churchill Livingstone.

ANSWER 35
A. TRUE B. TRUE C. TRUE D. FALSE E. FALSE

The foramen of munro connect the lateral and third ventricles

The third ventricle is a cavity of diencephalon

Refs:
Anatomy for Diagnostic Imaging. Ryan & McNicholas. W B Saunders Co Ltd.
Essential Anatomy by Lumley, Craven & Aitken. 3rd Edition, Churchill Livingstone.
Clinical Anatomy by Harold Ellis. 8th Edition. Churchill Livingstone.

ANSWER 36

A. FALSE   B. FALSE   C. TRUE   D. TRUE   E. TRUE

The superior sagittal sinus usually joins the right transverse sinus

The inferior sagittal sinus joins the straight sinus

Refs:
Anatomy for Diagnostic Imaging. Ryan & McNicholas. W B Saunders Co Ltd.
Essential Anatomy by Lumley, Craven & Aitken. 3rd Edition, Churchill Livingstone.
Clinical Anatomy by Harold Ellis. 8th Edition. Churchill Livingstone.

ANSWER 37

A. TRUE   B. FALSE   C. TRUE   D. FALSE   E. FALSE

The cochlea lies anterior to the vestibule

There are only five openings into the vestibules via three semicircular canals

Both saccule and utricle lie within the vestibule

Ref:
Anatomy for Diagnostic Imaging. Ryan & McNicholas. W B Saunders Co Ltd.
Essential Anatomy by Lumley, Craven & Aitken. 3rd Edition, Churchill Livingstone.
Clinical Anatomy by Harold Ellis. 8th Edition. Churchill Livingstone.

ANSWER 38

A. TRUE   B. TRUE   C. FALSE   D. TRUE   E. TRUE

The internal thoracic artery divides into musculophrenic and superior epigastric artery

Ref:
Anatomy for Diagnostic Imaging. Ryan & McNicholas. W B Saunders Co Ltd.
Essential Anatomy by Lumley, Craven & Aitken. 3rd Edition, Churchill Livingstone.
Clinical Anatomy by Harold Ellis. 8th Edition. Churchill Livingstone.

ANSWER 39

A. TRUE   B. TRUE   C. TRUE   D. FALSE   E. TRUE

The right paraspinal line is less than 2mm whereas the left can be up to 10mm

Ref:
Anatomy for Diagnostic Imaging. Ryan & McNicholas. W B Saunders Co Ltd.
Essential Anatomy by Lumley, Craven & Aitken. 3rd Edition, Churchill Livingstone.
Clinical Anatomy by Harold Ellis. 8th Edition. Churchill Livingstone.

ANSWER 40
A. FALSE   B. FALSE   C. FALSE   D. FALSE   E. TRUE

The vomer forms posteroinferior part of the septum

Only superior and middle conchae are part of the ethmoid bone, however the inferior concha is a separate bone

The floor of the maxillary sinus lies at a lower level than the floor of the nasal cavity

The perpendicular plate of palatine bone contributes to the lateral wall of the nasal cavity

Ref:
Anatomy for Diagnostic Imaging. Ryan & McNicholas. W B Saunders Co Ltd.
Essential Anatomy by Lumley, Craven & Aitken. 3rd Edition, Churchill Livingstone.
Clinical Anatomy by Harold Ellis. 8th Edition. Churchill Livingstone.

ANSWER 41
A. TRUE   B. FALSE   C. FALSE   D. TRUE   E. TRUE

To opacify the SVC simultaneous injection into both arms is required.

Clot dislodgement causing venous thrombosis is rarely reported.

Ref: Chapman & Nakielny. A Guide to Radiological Procedures. 3rd Edition. W B Saunders Co Ltd.

ANSWER 42
A. TRUE   B. FALSE   C. TRUE   D. FALSE   E. TRUE

BPD is most reliable in the second trimester. The yolk sac is reliably detected by TVS at 5.5 weeks.

Ref: Grainger & Allison. Diagnostic Radiology. 3rd Edition. Churchill Livingstone.

ANSWER 43
A. TRUE   B. FALSE   C. FALSE   D. TRUE   E. FALSE

Scarring will be detected with a Mag-3 renogram if renal function is good.

It allows assessment of divided renal function. 80% is actively secreted by proximal convoluted tubal, whilst 20% is filtered. Images are required from 0-30 minutes.

Ref: Chapman & Nakielny. A Guide to Radiological Procedures. 3rd Edition. W B Saunders Co Ltd.

ANSWER 44
A. TRUE   B. FALSE   C. TRUE   D. FALSE   E. TRUE

The patient needs to be fully conscious in order to describe pain. 0.5 - 1 ml of non-ionic contrast media is introduced into the nucleus pulposus, often followed by 0.2 - 0.3 ml of bupacaine. If the needle passes too anteriorly a major vessel can be punctured and cause retroperitoneal haemorrhage.

Ref: Chapman & Nakielny. A Guide to Radiological Procedures. 3rd Edition. W B Saunders Co Ltd.

ANSWER 45
A. TRUE   B. FALSE   C. TRUE   D. FALSE   E. FALSE

Ref: Bell and Finlay. Basic Radiographic Positioning and Anatomy. 1st Edition. Bailliere Tindall.

ANSWER 46
A. TRUE   B. FALSE   C. FALSE   D. FALSE   E. TRUE

CT has greater resolution than MRI. ^{75}Se-cholesterol is taken up by the adrenal cortex, and is used to demonstrate functioning cortical adenomas. ^{123}I-MIBG is taken up by the adrenal medulla and is used to demonstrate phaeochromocytomas.

Ref: Grainger & Allison. Diagnostic Radiology. 3rd Edition. Churchill Livingstone.

ANSWER 47
A. FALSE   B. TRUE   C. TRUE   D. FALSE   E. TRUE

Ref: Grainger & Allison. Diagnostic Radiology. 3rd Edition. Churchill Livingstone.

ANSWER 48
A. TRUE   B. TRUE   C. FALSE   D. TRUE   E. FALSE

The spleen is visualised during the arterial phase, while the liver is mainly visualised during the portall venous phase. Colloid shift is the increased distribution of isotope to the spleen and bone marrow indicating diffuse liver disease or portal hypertension.

Ref: Grainger & Allison. Diagnostic Radiology. 3rd Edition. Churchill Livingstone.

ANSWER 49
A. FALSE   B. TRUE   C. TRUE   D. TRUE   E. TRUE

A prolonged prothrombin time is not a contraindication.

Ref: Chapman & Nakielny. A Guide to Radiological Procedures. 3rd Edition. W B Saunders Co Ltd.

ANSWER 50
A. TRUE   B. FALSE   C. TRUE   D. FALSE   E. TRUE

Barium incites a reaction in the pleura. Following aspiration barium is usually coughed up but may need physiotherapy. Gastrograffin causes a severe chemical pneumonitis whilst gastromiro does not induce a reaction in lung parenchyma. Barium in serous cavities causes a marked inflammatory response leading to fibrosis.

Ref: Whitehouse & Worthington. Techniques in Diagnostic Imaging. 3rd Edition. Blackwell Science Ltd.

ANSWER 51
A. TRUE   B. FALSE   C. FALSE   D. FALSE   E. FALSE

Oesophageal symptons can be caused by stomach pathology

The upper oesophagus should only be imaged if symptoms suggest upper oesophagus lesion. To look for reflux turn patient from left side to right side. The mandatory projections are RAO or LAO erect and prone LPO.

Ref: Whitehouse & Worthington. Techniques in Diagnostic Imaging. 3rd Edition. Blackwell Science Ltd.

ANSWER 52

A. FALSE   B. TRUE   C. FALSE   D. TRUE   E. TRUE

The Barium barticles used for an enema are small particles 0.6-1.4 u and are coated to provide certain characteristics such as plasticity and rapid flow. Without antifoaming agents it cracks.

Ref: Whitehouse & Worthington. Techniques in Diagnostic Imaging. 3rd Edition. Blackwell Science Ltd.

ANSWER 53

A. FALSE   B. FALSE   C. FALSE   D. TRUE   E. TRUE

A 7.5 - 10 MHz transducer is required which can be rotated through 360 degrees. The stomach should be filled with de-aerated water.

Ref: Chapman & Nakielny. A Guide to Radiological Procedures. 3rd Edition. W B Saunders Co Ltd.

ANSWER 54

A. FALSE   B. FALSE   C. TRUE   D. FALSE   E. FALSE

A high speed rotation anode and a focal spot of 0.3-1.2 mm sq. are required. A tilting table top is desirable but most dedicated vascular suites do not have this facility. This is usually added on to a multipurpose digital unit nowadays.

Ref: Whitehouse & Worthington. Techniques in Diagnostic Imaging. 3rd Edition. Blackwell Science Ltd.

ANSWER 55

A. TRUE   B. TRUE   C. FALSE   D. FALSE   E. FALSE

Blood glucose levels should be checked in diabetics. ECG monitoring is ony required in patients with cardiac disease. No solids should be taken but fluids encouraged up to 2 hours before to avoid dehydration.

Ref: Chapman & Nakielny. A Guide to Radiological Procedures. 3rd Edition. W B Saunders Co Ltd.

ANSWER 56

A. TRUE   B. TRUE   C. TRUE   D. TRUE   E. FALSE

Either GE to look at the talar dome or STIR to look for bone marrow signal changes.

Ref: MRI in Orthopaedics and Sports Medicine. Stoller. Lippincott Raven.

ANSWER 57

A. FALSE   B. FALSE   C. FALSE   D. FALSE   E. TRUE

3-5 mls of contrast are injected (children 1-2 mls). Hip arthrography is a single contrast study. An anterior approach is standard. The joint is observed under passive movement.

Ref: Chapman & Nakielny. A Guide to Radiological Procedures. 3rd Edition. W B Saunders Co Ltd.

ANSWER 58

A. FALSE   B. TRUE   C. FALSE   D. FALSE   E. TRUE

The half time for ^{81m}Krypton is 13 sconds. The half life for ^{127}Xenon is 36.4 days and for ^{113m}Indium is 1000 seconds.

Ref: Chapman & Nakielny. A Guide to Radiological Procedures. 3rd Edition. W B Saunders Co Ltd.

ANSWER 59

A. FALSE   B. FALSE   C. FALSE   D. FALSE   E. TRUE

100 - 150 mls of non-ionic contrast media is required for an average adult injected at a rate of 3-5 mls per second. The scan starts below the level of the left atrium and moves cephalad. This is done as a single breathhold technique and therefore if the patient is breathless and starts breathing, it is likely to occur above the level of the hila where respiratory artefact is less of a problem. A high resolution algorithm is only used for HRCT. HRCT is recommended nowadays prior to the angiogram as this can look for other causes for the patients shortness of breath.

Ref: Grainger & Allison. Diagnostic Radiology. 3rd Edition. Churchill Livingstone.

ANSWER 60

A. TRUE   B. FALSE   C. FALSE   D. FALSE   E. FALSE

AP shoulder - coracoid process

Lateral toes - head of 1st metatarsal

Lateral foot - cubonavicular joint

Lateral view of the calcaneus - talocalcaneal joint

Bell and Finlay. Basic Radiographic Positioning and Anatomy. 1st Edition. Bailliere and Finlay.

Exam 6

QUESTION 1

Regarding silver recovery following film processing

A. In the electrolytic method silver is deposited as 90-95% pure metallic silver
B. In the electrolytic method silver is deposited on the anode
C. In the electrolytic method agitation of either the cathode or the anode serves no useful purpose
D. In the electrolytic method it is possible to recover silver from the wash water
E. The metallic replacement method is a more expensive procedure than the electrolytic method

QUESTION 2

Regarding image quality in image intensifier (II) systems

A. The spatial resolution (SR) of the II alone is about 4-5 lp/mm
B. When imaging with a 35mm film from the II, the SR is about 2 lp/mm
C. The SR of a TV camera system is about 1 lp/mm
D. Veiling glare is worse with larger sizes of II
E. A vidicon camera has a gamma of 0.8 whilst a plumbicon camera has a gamma of 1.0

QUESTION 3

The following statements are true

A. In fluoroscopy with an undercouch tube, drapes of at least 0.35mm lead equivalent are attached to the lower edge
B. In gamma imaging, body aprons should have at least 0.5mm lead equivalence
C. 2.5mm lead equivalence is often satisfactory for use in the walls, doors and windows of an x-ray room
D. 60mm of concrete is approximately equal to 1mm lead equivalence
E. 12mm of barium plaster is approximately equal to 1mm lead equivalence

QUESTION 4

The following statements regarding the characteristic curve are true

A. The characteristic curve (CC) is a graph of optical density (X-axis) vs relative exposure (Y-axis)
B. The part of the CC which relates to correct exposure is usually at the shoulder region of the curve
C. Film gamma refers to the area under the CC
D. In the solarization region of the CC, increasing the exposure further produces an increase in film density
E. Solarization film is usually used for film copying

QUESTION 5

The following are true

A. In Thompson scattering, photons are scattered with an associated change in energy
B. Compton scattering depends only on the number of electrons per unit mass
C. The probability of the photoelectric effect occuring increases with increasing photon energy
D. The Compton effect is dependent upon the atomic number (Z) of the material irradiated
E. The mass attenuation coefficient (MAC) is dependent upon both the linear attenuation coefficient (LAC) and the density of the material irradiated

QUESTION 6

Regarding radioactivity

A. Stable lighter radioactive nuclei contain nearly equal numbers of protons and neutrons
B. Stable heavy radioactive nuclei contain a greater proportion of neutrons than protons
C. Isotopes of an element are nuclides which have the same number of protons but differing number of neutrons
D. Isotopes of an element are nuclides which have the same chemical properties but differing physical properties
E. Isotopes of an element are nuclides which have the same position in the periodic table

QUESTION 7

Regarding ultrasound (U/S)

A. An U/S beam may be focused by using a convex piezoelectric element
B. The greater the curvature of a piezoelectric element, the longer the focal length
C. U/S may be focused using a plastic acoustic lens
D. U/S may be focused by using a curved mirror
E. Transducers with a short focal length, suffer from increased divergence of the far field

QUESTION 8

The following are non-stochastic effects

A. Cataract formation
B. Skin erythema
C. Sterility
D. Leukaemia
E. Muscular dystrophy

QUESTION 9

The following statements are true

A. Aliasing is an artefact of continuous wave Doppler
B. The Doppler effect is a change in the perceived frequency of sound emitted by a moving source
C. Maximum Doppler shift occurs when motion is at right angles to the transducer face
D. In order to produce continuous wave Doppler, a high Q transducer with no backing block is used
E. With continuous wave Doppler it is not possible to distinguish between flow in two overlapping vessels, at different depths in the beam

QUESTION 10

Which of the following interactions between x-rays and matter do not result in a change in energy of the incident photon

A. Pair production
B. Photodisintegration
C. Photoelectric effect
D. Coherent scattering
E. Compton scattering

QUESTION 11

Regarding atomic magnetism

A. Manganese^{3+} has been used a positive contrast media in MRI
B. Iron oxide is a super paramagnetic contrast media
C. Super-paramagnetic contrast media act by producing local magnetic field gradients
D. Super-paramagnetic contrast media shorten both T2$\star$ and T2
E. Super-paramagnetic contrast media are positive contrast agents

QUESTION 12

Regarding image quality in CT

A. For high contrast objects, the spatial resolution (SR) of a CT scanner approaches 5 lp/mm
B. For low contrast objects (1-2% contrast), an object may need to be 5-10mm in diameter before it can be resolved
C. Contrast in a structure is usually only detectable if its contrast is 10 times greater than the noise in the image
D. Contrast resolution in CT is 0.5%
E. "Bone algorithms" are used to enhance spatial resolution

QUESTION 13

In xeroradiography

A. Crystalline selenium is used
B. Pure selenium must be used
C. The selenium layer has a thickness of 130 microns
D. Has no advantages over conventional mammography
E. The developing process is dry and rapid

QUESTION 14

Regarding MRI

A. The time constant T2★ refers to the MR signal measured from free induction decay (FID)
B. T2★ results from non-uniformity of the static magnetic field
C. A spin echo sequence is used to remove the effect of the imperfections in the static magnetic field
D. In a spin echo sequence, a 90 degree pulse is followed by a 180 degree pulse, after which the signal is measured
E. In a spin echo sequence, the 90 degree pulse eliminates the dephasing effect of the magnetic field inhomogeneities

QUESTION 15

Regarding the half lives of radionuclides

A. The half life of ^{81m}Krypton is 13 seconds
B. The half life of ^{13}Nitrogen is 100 minutes
C. The half life of ^{11}Carbon is 200 minutes
D. The half life of ^{99}Technetium is 6 hours
E. The half life of ^{18}Fluorine is 112 minutes

QUESTION 16

Regarding MRI

A. In gradient recalled echo (GRE), the greater the tip angle the greater the T1 weighting
B. Chemical shift artefact occurs due to displacement in the frequency encoding direction
C. Chemical shift artefact can be reduced by using a steeper encoding gradient
D. The only technique currently available for MRA is "time of flight" angiography in GRE
E. The spatial resolution of MRI is two line pairs per millimetre

QUESTION 17

Regarding radionuclides and their principle uses

A. ^{111}Indium: Tumour detection
B. ^{67}Galium: Myocardial imaging
C. ^{67}Galium: Tumour detection
D. ^{81m}Kypton: Lung perfusion imaging
E. ^{201}Thalium: Myocardial perfusion imaging

QUESTION 18

The following are true regarding the equipment used in dental radiography

A. The total filtration of the beam should be equivalent to 2.5mm aluminium for xray tube voltages up to and including 70 kV
B. The xray tube voltage should not be lower than 50 kV and for intra-oral radiography should be preferably about 70 kV
C. The xray assembly should be marked to identify the nominal focal spot position
D. When using intra-oral film, a minimum focal spot to skin distance of not less than 20cm for equipment operating above 60 kV, is required
E. The exposure switch should be arranged so that the operator can be at least 1 metre away from the tube and the patient during exposure

QUESTION 19

Portable x-ray generators

A. A battery powered generator uses a battery which can store a charge equivalent to 10,000 mAs
B. In battery powered generators, the voltage does not fall between exposures
C. In battery powered generators the output from the transformer is single phase full wave rectified
D. A capacitor discharge generator is usually used in conjunction with a field emission x-ray tube
E. The advantage of a capacitor discharge generator is that it can deliver a large amount of power in an extremely short time

QUESTION 20

The following statements are true

A. In an xray tube, the total filtration should never be less than the equivalent of 0.5mm aluminium
B. For radiography of the chest, the focal spot to skin distance should not be less than 30cm
C. In hypocycloidal tomography and cerebral angiography, the use of lead or lead containing shields should be considered for protection of the lens of the patient's eye
D. During fluoroscopy, palpation with the hand should only be undertaken with an overcouch tube
E. A protective glove with a lead equivalent thickness of at least 0.25mm should be used for xrays up to 150 kV

QUESTION 21

The following statements are true

A. The normal atlanto-axial distance in a child is 5mm
B. The normal mandibular angle is 110 degrees in an adult
C. The third ventricle measures up to 7mm across in a coronal plane
D. The lowest foramen transversarium containing the vertebral artery at C5 is seen in 5% of cases
E. Hyperostosis frontalis interna is 10 times more common in women

QUESTION 22

Regarding normal variation

A. The coeliac axis and superior mesenteric artery arise from a common trunk in 0.5%
B. The left hepatic artery arises directly from the superior mesenteric artery in 10%
C. There is congenital absence of 1 kidney in approx 0.1% of cases
D. The splenic artery arises directly from the aorta in 0.5% of cases
E. The left renal vein is retro-aortic in 10% of cases

QUESTION 23

The following are true regarding fascia of the neck

A. The platysma is contained within the deep fascia of the neck
B. The pre-tracheal fascia is contained in the deep fascia
C. The cervical fascia encloses the sternocleidomastoid and trapezius muscles
D. The pre-vertebral fascia lies anterior to the brachial plexus
E. The carotid sheath encases the internal carotid artery medial to the internal jugular vein

QUESTION 24

The following are true

A. The cisterna chyli lies in front of the right crus of the diaphragm
B. The thoracic duct has many valves in its course
C. The right posterior intercostal arteries lie behind the thoracic duct
D. The thoracic duct in the neck passes behind the carotid vessels
E. The thoracic duct arches at the level of C7 over the left lung approximately 3-4cm below the clavicle

QUESTION 25

The following statements are true

A. The foramen lacerum is filled with fibrocartilage
B. The superior orbital fissures lies between greater and lesser wings of sphenoid
C. The foramen rotundum transmits the maxillary nerve
D. The foramen ovale is about 1.5cm in front of foramen rotundum
E. The hypoglossal canal lies posterior to the occipital condyle

QUESTION 26

Regarding the basal ganglia

A. The caudate nucleus and putamen form the corpus striatum
B. The head of the caudate nucleus is related to the anterior limb of internal capsule
C. The basal ganglia are supplied by striate branches of anterior and middle cerebral arteries
D. The main efferent pathway from the lentiform nucleus is via the globus palladus
E. The dentate nucleus is related to the posterior limb of the internal capsule

QUESTION 27

The following statements are true

A. The iliofemoral ligament is the strongest of the ligaments around the hip joint
B. The ischiofemoral ligament arises from the postero inferior margin of the acetabulum
C. The sciatic nerve supplies the hip joint
D. The femoral nerve lies medial to the femoral artery
E. The profunda femoris artery arises from the posteromedial aspect of the superficial femoral artery

QUESTION 28

The following are true

A. The base of the heart is mainly formed by left ventricle
B. The anterior surface of the heart is mainly formed by the right ventricle
C. The cavity of the right auricle lies to the left of the superior vena caval orifice
D. The right atrioventricular orifice lies to the right of inferior vena caval orifice
E. The inferior vena caval orifice is guarded by a thin fold of endocardium anteriorly

QUESTION 29

At the shoulder

A. The axillary vein lies lateral to the axillary artery
B. The glenoid labrum is deficient inferiorly
C. Subscapular muscle inserts into the lesser tuberosity of the humerus
D. The anterior circumflex humeral artery arises from the third part of the axillary artery
E. The acromioclavicular joint is a typical synovial joint

QUESTION 30

The following statements are true

A. Malrotation results in a left sided pancreas
B. Pancreatic tissue may completely surround the duodenum
C. Pancreas divisum occurs when the ventral and dorsal buds fail to fuse
D. The dorsal bud may fail to develop resulting in a pancreas with a head only
E. Accessory pancreatic nodules may occur within the stomach wall

QUESTION 31

The following statements are true

A. The os radiale externum is an accessory ossicle found distal to the radial styloid
B. In the majority of subjects, nutrient arteries enter the scaphoid in its distal half only
C. A metacarpal index of greater than 7.4 suggests arachnodactyly
D. The recessus sacciformis is a pouch anterior to the proximal radio-ulnar joint
E. The 1st carpo-metacarpal joint normally communicates freely with the 2nd carpo-metacarpal joint

QUESTION 32

The following are true

A. The nerve roots leave the cord anterolaterally and thus fore-shortened in AP view
B. In cervical myelography the cord occupies 25% of the interpedicular distance at C5/6
C. In CT of the spine the dorsal root ganglion may be seen
D. A single injection will normally opacify the anterior spinal artery
E. In MRI of the spine grey and white matter differentiation is not always possible

QUESTION 33

The following are true

A. The optic canal is entirely formed by the great wing of sphenoid
B. The ophthalmic artery lies inferior to the optic nerve in the optic canal
C. The optic canal transmits the superior ophthalmic vein
D. The optic canal connects the orbital apex with the suprasellar cistern
E. The intracranial portion of optic nerve is lateral to the internal carotid artery

QUESTION 34

The male urethra

A. Has a penile portion approximately 15 cm long
B. Has a dilated portion called the navicular fossa
C. The prostatic portion is the widest portion
D. The ejaculatory ducts open in the membranous urethra
E. Is partially lined with squamous epithelium

QUESTION 35

Regarding the radiographic features of the foot

A. Heel pad thickness is normally up to 24 mm in both sexes
B. Bohler's angle of the calcaneus is normally 30-35 degrees
C. The long axis of the talus is more horizontal in children under 5
D. The epiphysis of the styloid process of the 5th metatarsal may be mistaken for a fracture
E. The angle of the longitudinal arch of the foot normally measured 120-140 degrees

QUESTION 36

Following are true regarding the mid brain

A. The floor of the interpeduncular fossa is the anterior perforated substance
B. The inferior colliculus is joined to its respective optic tract
C. The medial geniculate body is connected to the optic tract
D. The part anterior to the cerebral aqueduct is called tectum or quadrigeminal plate
E. The cerebral aqueduct is always identified on a CT scan

QUESTION 37

The internal iliac artery

A. Divides into medial and lateral branches
B. Gives off the obturator artery near its origin
C. Gives off a branch which supplies the rectum
D. Arises anterior to the sacroiliac joint
E. Lies posterior to the internal iliac vein

QUESTION 38

The following statements are true

A. The normal thickness of the pericardium is 4-5mm
B. The transverse sinus lies anterior to the ascending aorta
C. The fat present between the epicardium and myocardium increases with age
D. The pericardium receives its blood supply from branches of the pulmonary arteries
E. Blood from the pericardium is drained to the azygous system

QUESTION 39

The gallbladder

A. Has a capacity of about 50 ml
B. Is related to the anterior abdominal wall
C. Is related to the first part of the duodenum
D. The cystic artery usually arises from the right hepatic artery
E. Is usually firmly attached to the posterior surface of the liver

QUESTION 40

The left suprarenal gland

A. Is a posterior relation of the body of the pancreas
B. Is covered with peritoneum of the greater sac
C. The left suprarenal vein drains into the inferior vena cava
D. Drains to para-aortic lymph nodes
E. Receives blood from the left inferior phrenic artery

QUESTION 41

The following statements are true of a DMSA renogram

A. DMSA allows detection of ectopic renal tissue
B. DMSA is excreted by glomerular filtration
C. Imaging should be performed immediately
D. A pelvic kidney is most well demonstrated by a posterior view
E. DMSA delivers a higher dose to the patient than Mag-3

QUESTION 42

Regarding percutaneous extraction of retained biliary calculae

A. Must be performed within one month of a T-tube cholangiogram
B. Has higher morbidity and mortality rates than endoscopic sphincterotomy
C. Is performed via the T-tube
D. Repeated attempts over several weeks may be required
E. Prophylactic antibiotics are required

QUESTION 43

The following tube angulations are correct

A. Axial view of calcaneus - 30 degrees of cranial angulation
B. Tunnel view of the knee - 110 degree angulation to the shaft of the tibia
C. Tunnel view of knee - 90 degree angulation to the shaft of the tibia
D. AP cervical spine - 5 degree cephalad
E. Submentovertex - 5 degrees cephalad

QUESTION 44
Ultrasound of the pylorus in infants

A. Muscle is hypoechoic
B. Mucosa is hyperechoic
C. The pyloric canal should be measured
D. A muscle thickness greater than 3 mms is abnormal
E. Pyloric volume is the best parameter

QUESTION 45
Regarding gestational dating

A. Spinal flexion may produce falsely low crown rump length values towards the end of the first trimester
B. The biparietal diameter is performed by measuring leading edge to leading edge of the skull vault
C. A transverse scan at the widest part of the skull demonstrates both thalami and the cavum septum pellucidum
D. The ratio of head circumference to abdominal circumference gives an accurate assessment of gestational age in the second trimester
E. The hyperechoic distal femoral point should be included in measurements of femur length

QUESTION 46
Dynamic spiral CT of the chest

A. Uses a high resolution algorithm
B. Requires 50 mls of non-ionic contrast media
C. An injection rate of 5 mls per second is routine
D. A pitch of 1 is recommended
E. A pitch of 1 represents one spiral scan covering 360 degrees

QUESTION 47
Lung biopsy

A. Is complicated by a pneumothorax in 50%
B. The patient should be turned onto the side of biopsy if a pneumothorax develops
C. A chest drain is necessary in 10% of pneumothoraces
D. Pneumothorax development is commoner in the prone position
E. Haemoptysis occurs in 1%

QUESTION 48
Regarding hysterosalpingograms

A. Prophylactic pain control is routine
B. Pethidine is an appropriate analgesic
C. A full bladder can cause pseudo obstruction of the fallopian tubes
D. Approximately 10 mls of warmed water-soluble contrast media is introduced into the uterine cavity
E. Cervical manipulation can induce syncope

QUESTION 49
Bowel preparation for barium enema

A. Bisocodyl
B. Castor oil
C. Calcium Citrate
D. Sodium picosulphate
E. Magnesium oxide

QUESTION 50
Regarding infusion rates of contrast during angiography

A. Aorta and legs - 10 mls per second
B. Coeliac axis angiography - 6 - 8 mls per second
C. Selective renal angiography 6-10 mls per second
D. IMA angiography - 5 mls per second
E. Carotid angiography - 5 mls per second

QUESTION 51
Angiographic unit staff must

A. Wear lead aprons with lead equivalent to 0.25 - 0.5 mm
B. Wear a whole-body radiation dose monitor
C. Wear a peripheral radiation dose monitor
D. Be immunised against Hep B virus
E. Wear a thyroid shield

QUESTION 52
Regarding ultrasound of the upper abdomen

A. The spleen is more echogenic than the liver in adults
B. The spleen is more echogenic than the renal cortex in adults
C. The renal sinus is more prominent in a neonate than an adult
D. The renal cortex is more echogenic than the spleen in a neonate
E. The renal cortex is more echogenic than the renal sinus in adults

QUESTION 53
The following values are appropriate

A. ^{81m}Krypton - 190 KeV
B. ^{133}Xenon - 171 KeV
C. ^{127}Xenon - 172 KeV
D. ^{127}Xenon - 390 KeV
E. ^{127}Xenon - 203 KeV

QUESTION 54
When performing a peroperative cholangiogram

A. 20 mls of 300 mg/ml water soluble contrast media should be used
B. The common bile duct should not exceed 8 mms in diameter
C. Glucagon causes relaxation of the Sphincter of Oddi
D. Free flow of contrast media into the duodenum should be demonstrated
E. Retrograde filling of the intra-hepatic ducts is normal

QUESTION 55
Shoulder CT Arthrography

A. 4-6 mls contrast is required
B. 8-12 mls air is required
C. Is performed supine
D. Scanning should be performed in arrested respiration
E. 3 cms continguous scans

QUESTION 56
The following are used in Isotope small bowel studies

A. ^{99m}Tc sulphur colloid
B. ^{99m}Tc pertechnetate
C. RBC labelled with ^{99m}Tc
D. ^{99m}Tc labelled albumin
E. ^{111}Indium labelled leucocytes

QUESTION 57
In dental radiography

A. The deciduous teeth should all be present by 2.5 years
B. The upper permanent teeth erupt 6-12 months prior to the lower
C. The normal adult has 8 permanent premolars and 12 permanent molars
D. There are normally 8 deciduous premolar teeth
E. Tooth enamel is the most radio-opaque tissue in the body

QUESTION 58
Barium as a contrast medium

A. EZM HD is 225 w/v
B. EZM HD comes as a suspension
C. EZM HD is diluted with 55 mls of water
D. Baritop comes as a suspension
E. Barium incites a reaction in the bronchial tree

QUESTION 59

Regarding routine MRI of the hip

A. Both hips are demonstrated on axial images
B. Both hips are demonstrated on sagittal images
C. Axial GE sequences are used
D. Coronal T1 sequences are used
E. Coronal STIR sequences are used

QUESTION 60

The following are true of transcranial ultrasound

A. The choroid plexus is echogenic
B. The corpus callosum is best identified on the sagittal oblique views
C. The choroid plexus is found in the lateral ventricles anterior to the caudothalamic notch
D. The cerebellar tonsils are not well demonstrated
E. A cavum septum pellucidum is a normal variant

Exam 6: Answers

ANSWER 1
A. TRUE   B. FALSE   C. FALSE   D. FALSE   E. FALSE

Pure metallic silver is deposited on the cathode

Agitation of either the cathode or the anode brings fresh silver ions closer to the surface of the cathode and increases the yield of pure metallic silver

It is not possible to recover silver using the electrolytic method however silver may be recovered from the wash water using the metallic replacement method

The electrolytic method requires electrical power whereas the metallic replacement method involves the use of steel wool only.

Hence the electrolytic method is considerably more expensive to perform

Ref: Curry & Thomas. Christensen's Physics of Diagnostic Radiology. 4th Edition. Williams & Wilkins (Europe) Ltd.

ANSWER 2
A. TRUE   B. TRUE   C. TRUE   D. TRUE   E. TRUE

But note that the SR decreases for an entire II system i.e. when used with a video camera system/photospot film

Veiling glare is due to scattering of light particularly in the output window of the image intensifier

Despite the gamma differences of the various cameras, the gamma value of a TV monitor system can be varied, up to 2.0, so that the contrast of the system as a whole, is increased

Ref: Farr & Allisy-Roberts. Physics for Medical Imaging. 1st Edition. W B Saunders Co Ltd.

ANSWER 3
A. FALSE   B. FALSE   C. TRUE   D. FALSE   E. TRUE

The drapes should have at least 0.5mm of lead equivalence

Body aprons used in diagnostic radiology are essentially ineffective against the higher photon energies encountered in nuclear medicine

120mm of concrete is approximately equal to 1mm lead equivalence

Ref: Farr & Allisy-Roberts. Physics for Medical Imaging. 1st Edition. W B Saunders Co Ltd.

ANSWER 4
A. FALSE   B. FALSE   C. FALSE   D. FALSE   E. TRUE

The CC is a graph of log relative exposure (X-axis) vs optical density (Y-axis)

The region of correct exposure relates to the straight line portion

Film gamma relates to the maximum slope of the straight line portion of the CC

In the solarization region, Increasing exposure results in decreased film density

Ref: Farr & Allisy-Roberts. Physics for Medical Imaging. 1st Edition. W B Saunders Co Ltd.

ANSWER 5
A. FALSE   B. FALSE   C. FALSE   D. FALSE   E. FALSE

In Thompson scattering, radiation undergoes a change in direction without a change in wavelength, and therefore no change in energy

Compton scattering depends on both the physical density and the electron density of the material irradiated

The probability of the photo-electric effect occuring is inversely proportional to the cube of the incident photon energy

The probability of the Compton effect occuring is independent of Z.

The MAC is independent of the density of an absorber.

Ref: Farr & Allisy-Roberts. Physics for Medical Imaging. 1st Edition. W B Saunders Co Ltd.

ANSWER 6
A. TRUE   B. TRUE   C. TRUE   D. TRUE   E. TRUE

Isotopes have the same atomic number but differing mass numbers

Ref: Farr & Allisy-Roberts. Physics for Medical Imaging. 1st Edition. W B Saunders Co Ltd.

ANSWER 7
A. FALSE   B. FALSE   C. TRUE   D. TRUE   E. TRUE

U/S can be focussed by a concave / spherical piezoelectric element

The greater the curvature, the shorter the focal length

Ref: Farr & Allisy-Roberts. Physics for Medical Imaging. 1st Edition. W B Saunders Co Ltd.

ANSWER 8
A. TRUE   B. TRUE   C. TRUE   D. FALSE   E. FALSE

Leukaemia is a stochastic effect

Muscular dystrophy is a genetically inherited condition

Ref: Farr & Allisy-Roberts. Physics for Medical Imaging. 1st Edition. W B Saunders Co Ltd.

ANSWER 9

A. FALSE   B. TRUE   C. FALSE   D. TRUE   E. TRUE

Continuous wave Doppler does not suffer from aliasing. This is an artefact of pulsed wave Doppler

At right angles, no Doppler effect is shown. Doppler shift becomes maximal at the most acute angle of incidence possible

Ref: Farr & Allisy-Roberts. Physics for Medical Imaging. 1st Edition. W B Saunders Co Ltd.

ANSWER 10

A. FALSE   B. FALSE   C. FALSE   D. TRUE   E. FALSE

Coherent scattering is scattering in which radiation undergoes a change in direction without a change in wave length, and therefore no change in energy

Ref: Armstrong: Lecture Notes on the Physics of Radiology. 1st Edition 1990. Clinical Press Ltd.

ANSWER 11

A. TRUE   B. TRUE   C. TRUE   D. TRUE   E. FALSE

Manganese^{3+} is paramagnetic with 5 unpaired electrons

Areas of uptake appear black and hence super paramagnetic contrast media are called negative contrast agents

Ref: Farr & Allisy-Roberts. Physics for Medical Imaging. 1st Edition. W B Saunders Co Ltd.

ANSWER 12

A. FALSE   B. TRUE   C. FALSE   D. TRUE   E. TRUE

High contrast objects: SR: - 1 lp/mm

Contrast needs to be 3-5 times greater than the noise in the image for it to be detectable

Bone algorithms enhance SR at the expense of increased noise

Ref: Farr & Allisy-Roberts. Physics for Medical Imaging. 1st Edition. W B Saunders Co Ltd.

ANSWER 13

A. FALSE   B. TRUE   C. TRUE   D. FALSE   E. TRUE

Amorphous selenium is used because it has the properties of a photoconductor

At a thickness of 130 microns, selenium shows a maximum sensitivity to x-rays in the diagnostic energy range

Edge enhancement occurs because the toner is attracted away from the low voltage side to the high voltage side of any boundary resulting in a sharp change in density

Ref: Curry & Thomas. Christensen's Physics of Diagnostic Radiology. 4th Edition. Williams & Wilkins (Europe) Ltd.

ANSWER 14

A. TRUE   B. TRUE   C. TRUE   D. TRUE   E. FALSE

SE: It is the 180 degree pulse which eliminates the dephasing effect of the magnetic field inhomogeneities

Ref: Farr & Allisy-Roberts. Physics for Medical Imaging. 1st Edition. W B Saunders Co Ltd.

ANSWER 15

A. TRUE   B. FALSE   C. FALSE   D. FALSE   E. TRUE

The half life of ^{13}N is 10 minutes

The half life of ^{11}C is 20 minutes

The half life of ^{99}Tc is 200,000 years. ^{99m}Tc has a half life of 6 hours

Ref: Farr & Allisy-Roberts. Physics for Medical Imaging. 1st Edition. W B Saunders Co Ltd.

ANSWER 16

A. TRUE   B. TRUE   C. TRUE   D. FALSE   E. FALSE

Phase contrast angiography is an additional method for performing MRA

The spatial resolution of MRI is about 0.5 line pairs per millimetre

Ref: Farr & Allisy-Roberts. Physics for Medical Imaging. 1st Edition. W B Saunders Co Ltd.

ANSWER 17

A. FALSE   B. FALSE   C. TRUE   D. FALSE   E. TRUE

^{111}Indium is used to label white cells for locating infective foci

^{81m}Krypton is used for lung ventilation studies

Ref: Farr & Allisy-Roberts. Physics for Medical Imaging. 1st Edition. W B Saunders Co Ltd.

ANSWER 18

A. FALSE   B. TRUE   C. TRUE   D. TRUE   E. FALSE

The total filtration of the beam should be equivalent to 1.5mm aluminium for xray tube voltages up to and including 70 kV, and 2.5mm aluminium of which 1.5mm should be permanent for xray tube voltages above 70 kV.

Every xray source assembly should be marked to identify the nominal focal spot position.

When using intra-oral film, the equipment should be provided with a field defining spacer cone which will ensure a minimum focal spot to skin distance of not less than 20cm for equipment operating above 60 kV and not less than 10cm for equipment operating at lower voltages.

For dental, mobile and portable equipment, the exposure switch should be arranged so that the operator can be at least 2 metres away from the tube and the patient during an exposure. For fixed equipment, the exposure switch should be located at the control panel.

Ref: AC1/185, AC2/7, Regulation 32, Regulation 8: IRR 88.

ANSWER 19

A. TRUE   B. FALSE   C. TRUE   D. TRUE   E. TRUE

Between exposures the voltage falls, and this drop needs to be compensated by recharging the battery from the mains

Ref: Armstrong: Lecture Note on the Physics of Radiology. 1st Edition. 1990. Clinical Press Ltd.

ANSWER 20

A. TRUE   B. FALSE   C. TRUE   D. FALSE   E. TRUE

The focal spot to skin distance should never be less than 30cm, and preferably not less than 45cm when stationary equipment is used. For radiography of the chest the distance should not be less than 60cm.

During fluoroscopy, palpation with the hand should be reduced to the minimum. It should only be undertaken on the image receptor side of the patient and therefore should not be carried out at all with an overcouch tube.

Ref: Regulation 12 and Regulation 6: IRR 88.

ANSWER 21

A. TRUE   B. TRUE   C. TRUE   D. TRUE   E. TRUE

Refs:
Anatomy for Diagnostic Imaging. Ryan & McNicholas. W B Saunders Co Ltd.
Essential Anatomy by Lumley, Craven & Aitken. 3rd Edition. Churchill Livingstone.
Clinical Anatomy by Harold Ellis. 8th Edition. Churchill Livingstone.

ANSWER 22

A. TRUE   B. FALSE   C. TRUE   D. TRUE   E. FALSE

The right hepatic artery arises from the SMA in 10%

The left renal vein is retroaortic in 3.5%

Refs:
Last's Anatomy. McMinn. 9th Edition. Churchill Livingstone.
Gray's Anatomy. 38th Edition. Churchill Livingstone.
An Atlas of Anatomy Basic to Radiology. Meschan. W B Saunders Co Ltd.

ANSWER 23

A. FALSE   B. TRUE   C. TRUE   D. TRUE   E. TRUE

The platysma is within the superficial fascia

Ref:
Anatomy for Diagnostic Imaging. Ryan & McNicholas. W B Saunders Co Ltd.
Essential Anatomy by Lumley, Craven & Aitken. 3rd Edition. Churchill Livingstone.
Clinical Anatomy by Harold Ellis. 8th Edition. Churchill Livingstone.

ANSWER 24

A. FALSE   B. TRUE   C. TRUE   D. TRUE   E. FALSE

The cisterna chyli lies behind the right crus of the diaphragm.

The thoracic duct arches over the left lung 3-4cm above the clavicle.

Refs:
Anatomy for Diagnostic Imaging. Ryan & McNicholas. W B Saunders Co Ltd.
Essential Anatomy by Lumley, Craven & Aitken. 3rd Edition. Churchill Livingstone.
Clinical Anatomy by Harold Ellis. 8th Edition. Churchill Livingstone.

ANSWER 25

A. TRUE   B. TRUE   C. TRUE   D. FALSE   E. FALSE

The foramen ovale is 1.5cm behind the foramen rotundum in the greater wing of sphenoid

The hypoglossal canal lies anterior and above the occipital condyle

Refs:
Anatomy for Diagnostic Imaging. Ryan & McNicholas. W B Saunders Co Ltd.
Essential Anatomy by Lumley, Craven & Aitken. 3rd Edition. Churchill Livingstone.
Clinical Anatomy by Harold Ellis. 8th Edition. Churchill Livingstone.

ANSWER 26

A. TRUE   B. TRUE   C. TRUE   D. TRUE   E. FALSE

Dentate nucleus is a part of cerebellum

Refs:
Anatomy for Diagnostic Imaging. Ryan & McNicholas. W B Saunders Co Ltd.
Essential Anatomy by Lumley, Craven & Aitken. 3rd Edition. Churchill Livingstone.
Clinical Anatomy by Harold Ellis. 8th Edition. Churchill Livingstone.

ANSWER 27

A. TRUE   B. TRUE   C. TRUE   D. FALSE   E. FALSE

The femoral nerve lies lateral to the femoral artery

The profunda femoris artery leaves the posterolateral aspect of the superficial femoral artery

Ref: Last's Anatomy. McMinn. 9th Edition. Churchill Livingstone.

ANSWER 28

A. FALSE   B. TRUE   C. TRUE   D. FALSE   E. TRUE

The base of the heart is mainly formed by the left atrium and its four pulmonary veins

The right atrioventicular orifice lies to the left of IVC orifice

Refs:
Anatomy for Diagnostic Imaging. Ryan & McNicholas. W B Saunders Co Ltd.

Essential Anatomy by Lumley, Craven & Aitken. 3rd Edition. Churchill Livingstone.
Clinical Anatomy by Harold Ellis. 8th Edition. Churchill Livingstone.

ANSWER 29
A. FALSE   B. FALSE   C. TRUE   D. TRUE   E. FALSE

The axillary vein lies medial to the axillary artery

The glenoid labrum is a continuous ring

The acromioclavicular joint is an atypical synovial joint

Refs:
Last's Anatomy. McMinn. 9th Edition. Churchill Livingstone.
Anatomy for Diagnostic Imaging. Ryan & McNicholas. W B Saunders Co Ltd.

ANSWER 30
A. FALSE   B. TRUE   C. TRUE   D. TRUE   E. TRUE

A left sided pancreas is an effect of laxity of the suspensory fascia

Refs:
Last's Anatomy. McMinn. 9th Edition. Churchill Livingstone.
Anatomy for diagnostic Imaging. Ryan & McNicholas. W B Saunders Co Ltd.

ANSWER 31
A. TRUE   B. FALSE   C. FALSE   D. FALSE   E. FALSE

In 13% of cases, nutrient arteries enter the scaphoid in its distal half only

A metacarpal index of greater than 8.4 suggests arachnodactyly

The recessus sacciformis is a pouch anterior to the distal radio-ulnar joint

The thumb carpo-metacarpal joint does not normally communicate with the 2nd carpo-metacarpal joint

Refs:
Last's Anatomy. McMinn. 9th Edition. Churchill Livingstone.
Gray's Anatomy. 38th Edition. Churchill Livingstone.
Anatomy for Diagnostic Imaging. Ryan & McNicholas. W B Saunders Co Ltd.

ANSWER 32
A. TRUE   B. FALSE   C. TRUE   D. FALSE   E. TRUE

The cord occupies 50-75% of the interpedicular distance.

Because the radicomedullary branches are segmental, multiple injections are required.

Refs:
Anatomy for Diagnostic Imaging. Ryan & McNicholas. W B Saunders Co Ltd.
Essential Anatomy by Lumley, Craven & Aitken. 3rd Edition. Churchill Livingstone.
Clinical Anatomy by Harold Ellis. 8th Edition. Churchill Livingstone.

ANSWER 33
A. FALSE   B. TRUE   C. FALSE   D. TRUE   E. FALSE

The optic canal is entirely formed by the lesser wing of sphenoid

Superior ophthalmic vein is transmitted through the superior orbital fissure

Intracranial portion of optic nerve is medial to the internal carotid artery

Refs:
Anatomy for Diagnostic Imaging. Ryan & McNicholas. W B Saunders Co Ltd.
Essential Anatomy by Lumley, Craven & Aitken. 3rd Edition. Churchill Livingstone.
Clinical Anatomy by Harold Ellis. 8th Edition. Churchill Livingstone.

ANSWER 34
A. TRUE   B. TRUE   C. TRUE   D. FALSE   E. TRUE

The ejaculatory ducts open in the prostatic urethra

Refs:
Last's Anatomy. McMinn. 9th Edition. Churchill Livingstone.
Gray's Anatomy. 38th Edition. Churchill Livingstone.
Anatomy for Diagnostic Imaging. Ryan & McNicholas. W B Saunders Co Ltd.

ANSWER 35
A. FALSE   B. TRUE   C. FALSE   D. TRUE   E. FALSE

Heel pad thickness: 21 mm in females. 23 mm in males

Long axis of the talus: It is more vertical in children under 5

The angle of the longitudinal arch of the foot is normally 130-170 degrees

Refs:
Last's Anatomy. McMinn. 9th Edition. Churchill Livingstone.
Anatomy for Diagnostic Imaging. Ryan & McNicholas. W B Saunders Co Ltd.

ANSWER 36
A. FALSE   B. FALSE   C. FALSE   D. FALSE   E. FALSE

The floor of the interpeduncular fossa is the posterior perforated substance

The inferior colliculus is joined to the auditory tract

The medial geniculate body is connected to the auditory tract

The tectum or quadrigeminal plate is posterior to the cerebral aqueduct

The cerebral aqueduct cannot always be identified on a CT scan.

Ref:
Anatomy for Diagnostic Imaging. Ryan & McNicholas. W B Saunders Co Ltd.
Essential Anatomy by Lumley, Craven & Aitken. 3rd Edition. Churchill Livingstone.
Clinical Anatomy by Harold Ellis. 8th Edition. Churchill Livingstone.

ANSWER 37

A. FALSE   B. FALSE   C. TRUE   D. TRUE   E. FALSE

The internal iliac artery divides into anterior and posterior divisions

The obturator artery is a branch of the anterior division

The internal iliac artery lies anterior to the internal iliac vein

Refs:
Last's Anatomy. McMinn. 9th Edition. Churchill Livingstone.
Anatomy for Diagnostic Imaging. Ryan & McNicholas. W B Saunders Co Ltd.

ANSWER 38

A. FALSE   B. FALSE   C. TRUE   D. FALSE   E. TRUE

Normal thickness of pericardium is 1-2mm only.

The transverse sinus lies behind the ascending aorta.

Pericardium receives its blood supply from branches of internal mammary artery.

Refs:
Anatomy for Diagnostic Imaging. Ryan & McNicholas. W B Saunders Co Ltd.
Essential Anatomy by Lumley, Craven & Aitken. 3rd Edition. Churchill Livingstone.
Clinical Anatomy by Harold Ellis. 8th Edition. Churchill Livingstone.

ANSWER 39

A. TRUE   B. TRUE   C. TRUE   D. TRUE   E. TRUE

Refs:
Last's Anatomy. McMinn. 9th Edition. Churchill Livingstone.
Anatomy for Diagnostic Imaging. Ryan & McNicholas. W B Saunders Co Ltd.

ANSWER 40

A. TRUE   B. FALSE   C. FALSE   D. TRUE   E. TRUE

The left suprarenal gland is covered with peritoneum on the lesser sac

The left suprarenal gland drains into the left renall vein

Ref: Last's Anatomy. McMinn. 9th Edition. Churchill Livingstone.

ANSWER 41

A. TRUE   B. FALSE   C. FALSE   D. FALSE   E. TRUE

DMSA is actively secreted by tubules

Imaging should not be performed before 1.5 hours in order to allow any free technitium to clear from the urinary tract. The anterior view is best to demonstrate a pelvic kidney.

Ref: Grainger & Allison. Diagnostic Radiology. 3rd Edition. Churchill Livingstone.

ANSWER 42
A. FALSE   B. FALSE   C. FALSE   D. TRUE   E. TRUE

Percutaneous extraction of a retained calculus should not be performed before at least one month. The procedure has lower morbidity and mortality than a sphincterotomy. The T-tube is removed and the procedure is performed via the fistulous tract.

Ref: Chapman & Nakielny. A Guide to Radiological Procedures. 3rd Edition. W B Saunders Co Ltd.

ANSWER 43
A. TRUE   B. TRUE   C. TRUE   D. FALSE   E. TRUE

110 degree angulation demonstrates the anterior aspect of the intercondylar notch

90 degree angulation demonstrates the posterior aspect of the intercondylar notch

AP cervical spine - 15 degrees cephalad

Ref: Bell and Finlay. Basic Radiographic Positioning and Anatomy. 1st Edition. Bailliere Tindall.

ANSWER 44
A. TRUE   B. TRUE   C. TRUE   D. FALSE   E. FALSE

The pyloric canal should be less than 15 mm in length and less than 3 mm in thickness. A thickness of greater than 5 mm is abnormal. 3 - 5 mm is equivocal. No universal agreement to which is the best parameter.

Ref: Chapman & Nakielny. A Guide to Radiological Procedures. 3rd Edition. W B Saunders Co Ltd.

ANSWER 45
A. TRUE   B. TRUE   C. TRUE   D. FALSE   E. FALSE

There is good correlation between the ratio of head circumference to abdominal circumference and intra-uterine growth in the third trimester.

Including the hyperechoic distal femoral point gives artefactual lengthening.

Ref: Grainger & Allison. Diagnostic Radiology. 3rd Edition. Churchill Livingstone.

ANSWER 46
A. FALSE   B. FALSE   C. FALSE   D. FALSE   E. TRUE

A high resolution algorithms are used for HRCT only. 100 - 150 mls of non-ionic contrast media is required and an injection rate of 2-3 mls per second is routine; 5 mls per second is for CT pulmonary angiography. A pitch of 1.5 - 2 can be used. The manufacturers state that there is no perceivable difference in image quality between a pitch of 1.5 and a pitch of 2.

Ref: Grainger & Allison. Diagnostic Radiology. 3rd Edition. Churchill Livingstone.

ANSWER 47
A. FALSE   B. TRUE   C. TRUE   D. FALSE   E. FALSE

15 - 35% of lung biopsies are complicated by apneumothorax. Depends on numerous factors although the incidence of pneumothoraces is obviously much greater if one uses CT to detect them. The benefits of the prone position is controversial but may reduce number of patients who need chest drains. Haemoptysis occurs in 2-5%.

Ref: Chapman & Nakielny. A Guide to Radiological Procedures. 3rd Edition. W B Saunders Co Ltd.

ANSWER 48
A. TRUE   B. FALSE   C. TRUE   D. TRUE   E. TRUE

Pethidine causes smooth muscle relaxation and delays delineation of the fallopian tubes

Ref: Whitehouse & Worthington. Techniques in Diagnostic Imaging. 3rd Edition. Blackwell Science Ltd.

ANSWER 49
A. TRUE   B. TRUE   C. FALSE   D. TRUE   E. TRUE

Magnesium oxide and sodium picosulphate are both found in picolax. Magnesium citrate is formed when picolax is powder dissolved in water.

Ref: Whitehouse & Worthington. Techniques in Diagnostic Imaging. 3rd Edition. Blackwell Science Ltd.

ANSWER 50
A. TRUE   B. TRUE   C. FALSE   D. FALSE   E. FALSE

Selective renal, IMA and carotid angiography are usually performed usung a hand injection, renals at 4-5 mls per second and IMAs and carotids at 3-4 mls per second.

Ref: Chapman & Nakielny. A Guide to Radiological Procedures. 3rd Edition. W B Saunders Co Ltd.

ANSWER 51
A. TRUE   B. TRUE   C. FALSE   D. TRUE   E. FALSE

Peripheral radiation dose monitors and thyroid shields are optional.

Ref: Whitehouse & Worthington. Techniques in Diagnostic Imaging. 3rd Edition. Blackwell Science Ltd.

ANSWER 52
A. FALSE   B. TRUE   C. FALSE   D. TRUE   E. FALSE

The liver is more echogenic than the spleen. The renal sinus is less prominent in a neonate than in an adult because of a paucity of fat. The renal cortex less echogenic than renal sinus.

Ref: Grainger & Allison. Diagnostic Radiology. 3rd Edition. Churchill Livingstone.

ANSWER 53
A. TRUE   B. FALSE   C. TRUE   D. FALSE   E. TRUE

^{133}Xenon emits 81 KeV, 171 KeV is ^{111}Indium. ^{127}Xenon emits at three energies - 172, 203 and 375 KeV.

Ref: Chapman & Nakielny. A Guide to Radiological Procedures. 3rd Edition. W B Saunders Co Ltd.

ANSWER 54
A. FALSE   B. FALSE   C. TRUE   D. TRUE   E. TRUE

150 mg/ml contrast media is used in order not to obscure filling defects. The CBD should not exceed 12 mms in diameter.

Ref: Whitehouse & Worthington. Techniques in Diagnostic Imaging. 3rd Edition. Blackwell Science Ltd.

ANSWER 55
A. FALSE   B. FALSE   C. TRUE   D. TRUE   E. TRUE

1-3 mls of contrast and 4-8 mls of air are injected. CT shoulder arthrograms are always double contrast. Arrested respiration stops respiratory artefact.

Ref: Chapman & Nakielny. A Guide to Radiological Procedures. 3rd Edition. W B Saunders Co Ltd.

ANSWER 56
A. TRUE   B. TRUE   C. TRUE   D. FALSE   E. TRUE

Sulphur colloid is used for detecting bleeding. Pertechnetate is used for detecting Meckels Diverticulum and ectopic gastric mucosa. Labelled red blood cells are used for detecting bleeding, and labelled white cells for inflammatory bowel disease. Labelled albumin is no longer used.

Ref: Whitehouse & Worthington. Techniques in Diagnostic Imaging. 3rd Edition. Blackwell Science Ltd.

ANSWER 57
A. TRUE   B. FALSE   C. TRUE   D. FALSE   E. TRUE

The lower permanent teeth erupt 6-12 months earlier than the upper permanent teeth. There are no deciduous premolar teeth.

Ref: Grainger & Allison. Diagnostic Radiology. 3rd Edition. Churchill Livingstone.

ANSWER 58
A. FALSE   B. FALSE   C. FALSE   D. TRUE   E. FALSE

EZM HD comes as a powder form which is reconstituted with 60 mls water exactly to form a 250 w/v. Baritop comes as a suspension in a 300 ml can. Barium does not incite a reaction in the bronchial tree.

Ref: *Whitehouse & Worthington. Techniques in Diagnostic Imaging. 3rd Edition. Blackwell Science Ltd.*

ANSWER 59

A. TRUE   B. FALSE   C. FALSE   D. TRUE   E. TRUE

Only the symptomatic hip is demonstrated on the sagittal images. Axial T1, T2 and/or STIR sequences are usually performed.

Ref: *MRI in Orthopaedics and Sports Medicine. Stoller. Lippincott Raven.*

ANSWER 60

A. TRUE   B. FALSE   C. FALSE   D. TRUE   E. TRUE

The copus callosum is best identified on the midline sagittal views. The normal choroid plexus does not extend anterior to the caudothalamic notch.

Ref: *Grainger & Allison. Diagnostic Radiology. 3rd Edition. Churchill Livingstone.*

Exam 7

QUESTION 1
Regarding geometry of the x-ray image

A. Sharpness is the ability of an x-ray film screen system to define an edge
B. Sharpness is independent of the contrast of an image
C. Parallax is seen with single emulsion films
D. Absorption unsharpness is greatest for round or oval objects without sharp edges
E. Absorption unsharpness is greatest for coned shaped objects

QUESTION 2
Regarding scintillation counters

A. Sodium iodide may be used as a scintillation phosphor
B. Crystals of potassium iodide may be used as a scintillation phosphor
C. Crystals of anthracene and naphthalene may be used as scintillation phosphors
D. Scintillation counters cannot distinguish between radiations of different energies
E. A scintillation counter has both a longer dead time and a lower detection efficiency of radiation compared to Geiger Muller tubes

QUESTION 3
Regarding subject contrast

A. This refers to the difference in the intensity of transmitted radiation between one part of a subject compared to another part
B. The photoelectric effect is the most important contributor to subject contrast in diagnostic radiology
C. Higher kVp x-rays produce greater subject contrast than lower kVp x-rays
D. Low kVp exposures only permit a narrow exposure latitude
E. Contrast media do not play a role in subject contrast

QUESTION 4

Regarding the apparatus required for digital subtraction angiography

A. Specially designed x-ray tubes are required
B. The x-ray generator should be able to provide three phase voltage pulses and 12 pulses per cycle
C. A focal spot of 0.3 mm is desirable
D. A high quality image intensifier is needed
E. The x-ray tube should incorporate a high speed rotating anode

QUESTION 5

Regarding x-ray production

A. It is the deceleration of the electrons bombarding the target that results in the production of x-rays
B. X-radiation is produced by the processes of bremsstrahlung and characteristic radiation
C. The anode heel effect is more noticeable on large size x-ray film
D. A stationary anode tube has better cooling characteristics than a rotating anode one
E. A lower atomic number target produces an x-ray beam of greater intensity than a higher atomic numbered target

QUESTION 6

Regarding rotating anode tubes

A. Energy efficiency is much greater than in stationary anode tubes
B. The tube loading characteristics are greater as heat is generated over a focal track
C. The principal heat path is via radiation across the tube vacuum
D. The induction motor is situated inside the glass envelope to ensure maximum efficiency of the tube
E. The anode has a molybdenum stem backing in order to minimise heat conduction to the rotor mechanism

QUESTION 7

The following are the main parameters determined in MRI

A. T1
B. Spin Echo
C. GRASS
D. Proton density
E. T2

QUESTION 8

The following are criteria for attaining a radiograph of satisfactory quality

A. The density is controlled primarily by kV
B. Contrast is controlled primarily by mA
C. Ideally there should be minimum sharpness whilst maintaining the true outline of the image
D. Ideally there should be maximum sharpness whilst maintaining the true outline of the image
E. Film blackness is primarily controlled by mA

QUESTION 9

The following statements are true

A. Film gamma and exposure latitude are directly related
B. High gamma films have a narrow exposure latitude
C. The useful density range of a film is usually 0.25 - 2.0 above base + fog values
D. Typically wide latitude film is needed in mammography
E. The gamma of a film depends on the average size of the crystals in the film

QUESTION 10

The following statements regarding fluoroscopy are true

A. Quantum mottle is noticeable in both fluoroscopy and radiography
B. Noise reduces the perceptibility of structures having high contrast
C. For a structure to be detectable, its contrast must be at least 10 times the noise relative to the signal
D. Image quality in the less bright areas of an image is limited by noise
E. Spatial resolution improves with structures of higher contrast

QUESTION 11

Digital imaging

A. A 10 bit computer contains 2048 grey scale levels
B. The eye can only distinguish 32 grey scale levels
C. "Background subtraction" can be used to reduce the effect of scatter and veiling glare
D. Signal to noise ratio is improved by frame averaging
E. Noise reduction may be achieved by "high pass spatial filtering"

QUESTION 12

Regarding collimators used in gamma imaging

A. In a parallel hole collimator, the field of view and sensitivity vary with distance from the collimator face
B. A divergent hole collimator minifies an image
C. A convergent collimator minifies an image
D. A pinhole collimator magnifies an image
E. Both convergent and divergent collimators do not suffer from geometric distortion

QUESTION 13

Regarding Single Photon Emission Computed Tomography (SPECT)

A. Images acquired without filtered back projection show STAR artefacts
B. Images have a better spatial resolution than PET images
C. Attenuation correction is applied to take into account the shape of a patient
D. Attenuation correction is usually applied post-processing
E. Image data is acquired over 180 degrees when imaging the myocardium using thallium - 201

QUESTION 14

Regarding tissue weighting factors (Wt)

A. Gonads: Wt 0.2
B. Red bone marrow: Wt 0.12
C. Breast: Wt 0.12
D. Lung: Wt 0.05
E. Thyroid: Wt 0.05

QUESTION 15

Regarding dosimetry

A. Lithium fluoride (LiF) may be used as the phosphor material in a thermoluminescent dosemeter (TLD)
B. TLDs are suitable for finger dosimetry
C. When using film badges it is not possible to identify the type and energy of an exposure
D. LiF chips are annealed in order to remove any residual stored energy from a previous exposure
E. TLDs are not affective over a wide range of exposure doses

QUESTION 16

Regarding ultrasound (U/S)

A. In the absence of a matching plate, only approximately 20% of sound energy would be transmitted at a soft tissue - piezoelectric crystal interface
B. A matching plate, a quarter of a wavelength thick, is attached to the front of a transducer in order to prevent mismatch between soft tissue and the transducer
C. As little as 1% reflection of sound energy at an interface is detectable
D. Attenuation of U/S is measured in decibels (dB)
E. Sound energy is attenuated linearly with increasing depth of travel

QUESTION 17

Regarding ultrasound (U/S)

A. The Nyquist frequency is equal to half the pulse repetition frequency
B. In colour flow Doppler, flow away from the transducer is usually manifest as the colour red
C. A Cardiff test object can be used as a phantom in U/S quality assurance
D. The time averaged intensity of an U/S beam should not exceed 100 milliwatts (mW) per square centimetre
E. In physiotherapy, a typical U/S intensity used may be 1,000 mW per square centimetre

QUESTION 18

Regarding MRI

A. Water and CSF appear dark on T2 weighted images
B. In proton density weighted imaging, a time for repetition (TR) of 300-800 ms is typically used
C. Generally speaking, proton density weighting produces images with a small signal to noise ratio
D. In proton density weighted imaging, image contrast is principally due to differences in T1 relaxation properties of the tissues
E. CSF and fat appear bright on proton density weighted imaging

QUESTION 19

Signal to noise ratio in MRI can be increased by

A. Increasing the tip angle
B. Decreasing the band width of the receiving coils
C. Decreasing slice thickness
D. Using spin echo rather than gradient recalled echo (GRE)
E. Using well positioned surface coils

QUESTION 20

The following statements are true

A. The inherent filtration of every tube assembly should be marked permanently and clearly on the tube housing
B. For normal diagnostic work, the total filtration of the beam should be equivalent to not less than 2.5mm of aluminium of which 1.5mm should be permanent
C. All radiographic xray equipment should be provided with properly aligned adjustable beam limiting devices to keep the radiation beam within the limits of the xray film selected for each examination
D. The housing and supporting plates of an xray image intensifier should provide shielding equivalent of least 1mm lead for 100 kV
E. In mammography, the total permanent filtration should never be less than 0.3mm molybdenum

QUESTION 21

Regarding the cerebellum

A. It is connected by three pairs of cerebellar peduncles to the brain stem
B. The tonsils are the most inferior part of the cerebellar hemisphere
C. The anterior inferior cerebellar artery and the superior cerebellar artery arises from the basilar artery
D. The deepest fissure is the primary fissure at the superior surface
E. A CT of the upper cerebellum contains cerebellum posteriorly and occipital lobes antero-laterally

QUESTION 22

The following statements are true regarding the talus

A. It is the largest of the tarsal bones
B. It starts to ossify in the 9th fetal month
C. The lateral tubercle is the most posterior part of the talus
D. The medial and lateral tubercles are separated by a groove for flexor hallucis longus
E. The neck is grooved inferiorly as the sulcus tarsi

QUESTION 23

Regarding the knee

A. The posterior cruciate ligament is attached to the lateral femoral condyle
B. The anterior cruciate ligament prevents backward displacement of the tibia
C. The semimembranosus bursa communicates directly with the knee joint
D. The cruciate ligaments are of high signal on T1 weighted MRI scans
E. The ossification centre for the patella appears at 3 years

QUESTION 24

Regarding wrist and hand radiography

A. Two views are sufficient if scaphoid injury is suspected
B. The left hand is usually used for bone age
C. The distal radial articulation is angled about 12 degrees in the volar direction
D. The radial and ulnar styloid processes should be superimposed on a lateral wrist radiograph
E. A clenched fist view can be used to assess carpal instability

QUESTION 25

At mid-humerus level

A. The profunda brachii vessels lie lateral to the humerus
B. The brachial artery lies lateral to the median nerve
C. The basilic vein perforates the deep fascia of the arm
D. The radial nerve lies medial to the humerus
E. The brachial artery lies in contact with the humerus

QUESTION 26

Regarding the walls of the pelvis

A. Piriformis extends from the middle three sacral segments
B. Obturator internus arises from the bony margins of the obturator foramen
C. The obturator artery passes through the obturator canal below the obturator membrane
D. The sacral plexus is directly related to piriformis
E. Coccygeus (Ischiococcygeus) muscle lies above piriformis

QUESTION 27

The ovaries

A. Are supplied by a branch of the external iliac artery
B. Drain lymph to para-aortic nodes
C. Are covered by peritoneum
D. Measure approx. 2 cm in diameter
E. Attach to the uterus by the suspensory ligament of the uterus

QUESTION 28

The abdominal aorta

A. Starts at the level of T10 vertebra
B. Is crossed anteriorly by the splenic vein
C. Gives off suprarenal branches on both sides
D. Gives off the interior phrenic arteries at its commencement
E. Gives off the inferior epigastric artery at its bifurcation

QUESTION 29

Regarding the gallbladder (GB)

A. The neck is related to the lesser omentum
B. It is absent in 0.5% of cases
C. The neck contains spiral folds of mucosa
D. It may be double in 1% of cases
E. It may have a mesentery

QUESTION 30

Regarding lymphatic drainage

A. The gallbladder drains to nodes around the porta hepatis
B. The posterior abdominal wall drains to para-aortic nodes
C. The bare area of the liver drains to coeliac nodes
D. The inferior surface of the diaphragm drains to pre-aortic nodes
E. The lower oesophagus drains to coeliac nodes

QUESTION 31

The inferior vena cava

A. Has a longer course than the aorta in the abdomen
B. Begins at the level of the fifth lumbar vertebrae
C. Receives the inferior epigastric veins
D. Is crossed by the root of the ileal mesentery
E. Is closely related to the first part of the duodenum

QUESTION 32

The following statements are true

A. Of the 12 pairs of ribs 7 are true, 4 are false and 1 is floating
B. Each typical rib has 2 facets, 1 articulating with the same vertebral level and the 1 with the vertebra below
C. The costovertebral and costotransverse joints of a typical rib are of synovial type
D. The first rib is grooved posteriorly by the subclavian vein
E. The scalenus anterior muscle is attached to first and second ribs

QUESTION 33

Regarding the right atrium

A. Its anterior wall is smooth and into which the great vein drains
B. The coronary sinus drains into right atrium between the orifice of the IVC and the tricuspid valve
C. The fossa ovalis is an oval depression on the upper part of the inter-atrial septum
D. The crista terminalis separates the right atrium from its appendage
E. The posterior wall is smoother when compared to its anterior wall

QUESTION 34

The following are true

A. The cisterna chyli is anterior to the bodies of L1 and L2
B. The thoracic duct passes through the diaphragm at level T10
C. The terminal parts of hemi azygous system passes behind the thoracic duct to enter the azygous vein
D. The right lymphatic duct is about 5cm long
E. The normal length of thoracic duct is 25cm

QUESTION 35

The following are true

A. The cricoid cartilage forms a complete ring in transverse section
B. The true vocal cords lie inferior to the cricothyroid membrane
C. The aryepiglottic folds move towards each other during swallowing
D. The true vocal cords are adducted during gentle respiration
E. The epiglottis commonly calcifies in the adult

QUESTION 36

The following statements are true

A. Sternocleidomastoid has one head attached to the medial half of the clavicle
B. The scalenus anterior is attached superiorly to the anterior tubercles of lower three cervical vertebrae
C. The phrenic nerve lies posterior to scalenus anterior
D. The scalenus medius is attached inferiorly to the second rib
E. There are five pairs of strap muscles lying anteriorly in the neck

QUESTION 37

Regarding the cranial nerves

A. The third cranial nerve has both somatic motor and sensory fibres
B. The ciliary ganglion lies lateral to the optic nerve within the orbit
C. The fourth cranial nerve enters the orbit through the inferior orbital fissure
D. The fifth cranial nerve has a large sensory and smaller motor root
E. The sixth nerve passes through the cavernous sinus lateral to the internal carotid artery

QUESTION 38

Regarding the aorta

A. The ascending aorta is about 10cm long
B. The right pulmonary artery is posterior to the lower part of ascending aorta
C. The right main bronchus lies anterior to the lower part of the ascending aorta
D. The left vagus nerve lies anterior to the descending aorta
E. The left recurrent laryngeal nerve passes upwards posterior to the arch of aorta

QUESTION 39

The following are ectodermal in origin

A. Mouth
B. Lower anal canal
C. Membranous labyrinth
D. Ciliary body and iris
E. Tympanic antrum

QUESTION 40

Regarding the mandible

A. It is in contact with lingual nerve
B. It gives attachment to the sphenomandibular ligament at the lingula
C. It ossifies in membrane
D. It is retracted by the horizontal fibres of temporalis
E. It arises from the second pharyngeal arch

QUESTION 41
Regarding urethrography

A. The prostatic urethra is best demonstrated during micturation
B. Filling of cowpers gland is a normal finding
C. An ascending urethrogram demonstrates anatomy well up to the internal sphinctre
D. The foley catheter balloon is inflated in the fossa navalis during an ascending urethrogram
E. The bladder volume increases by approximately 80 mls per annum in a child

QUESTION 42
Regarding renal ultrasonography

A. Renal length is accurate to within 1 cm (approximately 10%) in 95% of cases
B. The renal cortex is thicker medially than laterally
C. The cortical thickness is that between the renal capsule and the outer aspect of the medullary pyramid
D. The cortical thickness is that between the renal capsule and the margin of the sinus echoes
E. The normal kidney is hypoechoic to liver or spleen

QUESTION 43
The following are true

A. An intravenous pyelogram is contraindicated within 48 hours of birth
B. A direct radionuclide micturating cystogram gives a ten fold lower dose than a radiographic micturating cystogram
C. A direct radionuclide micturating cystogram is less sensitive than a radiographic micturating cystogram at detecting vesicoureteric reflux
D. An indirect radionuclide micturating cystogram is performed 1-2 hours following an injection of ^{99m}Tc-labelled Mag 3 or ^{99m}Tc-labelled DTPA
E. Indirect micturating cystogram is more sensitive than a radiographic micturating cystogram at demonstrating reflux during voiding

QUESTION 44
Regarding oral cholangiography

A. An erect film is useful to demonstrate floating gallstones
B. Gallbladder contractility is evaluated by giving a fatty meal
C. Nonopacification of the gallbladder is diagnostic of chronic cholecystitis
D. A preliminary film is mandatory
E. Pseudalbuminuria is a side effect

QUESTION 45

Regarding abdominal ultrasound

A. Following cholecystectomy, the common bile duct can measure up to 1.5 cm
B. The cystic duct is visible in approximately 50%
C. The pancreatic duct usually measures less on ultrasound than at ERCP
D. The upper limit of normal for the pancreatic duct is 3.5 mm in diameter
E. The intraductal transducers have frequencies of 7.5-12 MHz

QUESTION 46

Regarding biopsy of the liver

A. Paracentesis should be performed prior to a percutaneous liver biopsy
B. A percutaneous liver biopsy should be performed in arrested respiration
C. A transvenous large cutting needle biopsy is contraindicated if there is a bleeding diaphysis
D. A plugged biopsy requires direct visualisation of the liver capsule
E. A brush biopsy can be performed via a T-tube catheter

QUESTION 47

The following are true of imaging the pancreas

A. Water is an appropriate oral contrast media for CT
B. The pancreas parenchyma enhances maximally during the portal venous phase
C. The normal duct measures up to 2 mm in diameter in the body of the pancreas on ultrasound
D. The normal duct measures up to 6.5 mms at the head of the pancreas at ERCP
E. The number of side branches of the pancreatic duct opacifying at ERCP decreases with age

QUESTION 48

When performing an orthopantomogram

A. Only the x-ray tube moves
B. The film cassette and x-ray tube move in opposite directions
C. The film is in a curved cassette
D. The cervical spine is demonstrated three times
E. The arc of rotation of the x-ray tube and film is always circular

QUESTION 49

Barium Swallow - Dynamic studies

A. Cine has higher radiation dose than rapid serial roll film
B. Cine has lower frame rate than rapid serial roll film
C. Should always be performed as part of routine barium swallow
D. Speed of 5 frames per second is sufficient
E. Multiple boluses of contrast should be given at any one time

QUESTION 50

Endoscopic Ultrasound

A. Is performed via an end view scope
B. Uses a mechanical sector probe
C. The scope has a rigid end
D. The patient lies on their right side
E. Orientation is dependant on distance from incisors

QUESTION 51

Double contrast barium enema - Technique

A. Run barium initially in right lateral position
B. Filling should be continued to the mid-transverse colon
C. Fill caecum in right lateral position
D. Turn patient around twice
E. Air insufflation in supine position

QUESTION 52

Nuclear Medicine gastro-oesophageal reflux studies in infants

A. Normal milk feed used
B. Tracer given before feed
C. Infant is placed in a right lateral decubitus position
D. Dynamic imaging for 30 - 60 minutes
E. Four hour images are performed

QUESTION 53

The following are true regarding vascular guide wires

A. The size is measured by the diameter
B. The diameter is in cms
C. Standard adult wire is a 0.035
D. Standard paediatric wire is 0.018
E. Standard interventional wire is 0.038

QUESTION 54

IV DSA

A. Uses larger volumes of contrast than intra-arterial studies
B. Uses a higher concentration of contrast than intra-arterial studies
C. Has a lower rate of contrast reactions than intra-arterial studies
D. Must be injected through a central line
E. Should have ECG monitoring

QUESTION 55
Routine MRI of the knee includes

A. True sagittal views
B. Volume coronal sequences
C. Axial sequences
D. Sagittal obliques
E. Axial images showing both knees

QUESTION 56
Wrist Arthrography

A. 2-4 mls contrast is required
B. 2-4 mls air is required
C. The wrist should be flexed 10-15 degrees
D. Injection site is the mid carpal region
E. Early views should be taken

QUESTION 57
Pulmonary angiography

A. Is contraindicated with a mean PA pressure of >30 mm of Hg
B. A mean PA pressure of 10 is normal
C. Requires a pigtail catheter
D. Requires a vascular sheath
E. Puncture the most easily palpable pulse

QUESTION 58
Radiopharmaceuticals for lung perfusion studies - the following statements are true

A. 5-20 nm particles used
B. Albumin particles can be used
C. Carbon particles can be used
D. Drawing blood into syringe can cause clumping
E. Particles occludes small lung vessels

QUESTION 59
Contraindications to V/Q scanning include

A. Severe heart failure
B. Left to right cardiac shunt
C. Severe pulmonary hypertension
D. Bleeding diathesis
E. Asthma

QUESTION 60

HRCT Lungs

- A. Windowing is centered at + 40 HU
- B. A window width of 1600 HU is used
- C. The dose from a 1 mm section is less than a 2 mm section
- D. The same collimation is used for a 1 mm and 2 mm slice
- E. Expiration scans are helpful

Exam 7: Answers

ANSWER 1
A. TRUE   B. FALSE   C. FALSE   D. TRUE   E. FALSE

Sharpness is dependent on the contrast of an image. An unsharp edge can easily be seen if contrast is high, conversely a sharp edge may be poorly seen if the contrast is low

Parallax only occurs with double emulsion films

Absorption unsharpness is least for coned shaped objects

Ref: Curry & Thomas. Christensen's Physics of Diagnostic Radiology. 4th Edition. Williams & Wilkins (Europe) Ltd.

ANSWER 2
A. TRUE   B. TRUE   C. TRUE   D. FALSE   E. FALSE

Scintillation counters are able to distinguish between radiations of different energies (unlike GM tubes)

There is less dead time and a higher detection efficiency than GM tubes

Ref: Armstrong. Lecture Notes on the Physics of Radiology. 1st Edition. 1990. Clinical Press Ltd.

ANSWER 3
A. TRUE   B. TRUE   C. FALSE   D. TRUE   E. FALSE

Low kVp x-rays produce greater subject contrast as more of the primary beam will be attenuated at the lower beam energies

Contrast media are of relatively high atomic number and therefore enhance subject contrast due to the photoelectric effect

Ref: Armstrong. Lecture Notes on the Physics of Radiology. 1st Edition 1990. Clinical Press Ltd.

ANSWER 4
A. FALSE   B. TRUE   C. FALSE   D. TRUE   E. TRUE

No special tubes are required, those already in use are usually suitable

It is undesirable to have a very small focal spot as this reduces tube loading. In addition the focal spot size in angiography is not a limiting factor to resolution. A focal spot size of 0.6 mm is adequate. 0.3 mm is usually necessary for macro angiography

High speed anodes are energized with three phase mains and rotate at about 9000 or 17000 rpm

Ref: Curry & Thomas. Christensen's Physics of Diagnostic Radiology. 4th Edition. Williams & Wilkins (Europe) Ltd.

ANSWER 5

A. TRUE   B. TRUE   C. TRUE   D. FALSE   E. FALSE

The intensity of the x-ray beam produced that passes through the anode is less than that towards the cathode. Hence with large size x-ray films the heel effect may be visible

The rotating anode tube has better cooling characteristics as the heat is spread over a larger target area

Higher atomic number elements are able to produce higher intensity x-ray beams. Hence tungsten, with it atomic number of 74, is an ideal target material

Ref: Armstrong. Lecture Notes on the Physics of Radiology. 1st Edition. 1990. Clinical Press Ltd.

ANSWER 6

A. FALSE   B. TRUE   C. TRUE   D. FALSE   E. TRUE

The energy conversion between both a rotating and stationary anode tube is identical. 99% of the energy goes towards heat production and only 1% towards x-ray production

The induction motor is situated outside the glass envelope within the insulating oil

Ref: Curry & Thomas. Christensen's Physics of Diagnostic Radiology. 4th Edition. Williams & Wilkins (Europe) Ltd.

ANSWER 7

A. TRUE   B. FALSE   C. FALSE   D. TRUE   E. TRUE

Spin Echo and GRASS are MRI sequences. The latter is a gradient echo sequence

Ref: Armstrong. Lecture Notes on the Physics of Radiology. 1st Edition. Clinical Press.

ANSWER 8

A. TRUE   B. FALSE   C. FALSE   D. TRUE   E. TRUE

The density, and as a consequence the contrast, is primarily controlled by kV

Ref: Curry & Thomas. Christensen's Physics of Diagnostic Radiology. 4th Edition. Williams & Wilkins (Europe) Ltd.

ANSWER 9

A. FALSE   B. TRUE   C. TRUE   D. FALSE   E. FALSE

Film gamma and exposure latitude are inversely related

High gamma, narrow latitude films are needed in mammography

The gamma of a film depends on the range of crystal sizes

Ref: Farr & Allisy-Roberts. Physics for Medical Imaging. 1st Edition. W B Saunders Co Ltd.

ANSWER 10
A. FALSE   B. FALSE   C. FALSE   D. TRUE   E. TRUE

Noise is not noticeable in radiography

Noise mainly affects low contrast structures

Contrast needs to be 2-5 times the noise relative to the signal, i.e. a 1mm structure will be seen if its contrast is at least 5%

Ref: Farr & Allisy-Roberts. Physics for Medical Imaging. 1st Edition. W B Saunders Co Ltd.

ANSWER 11
A. FALSE   B. TRUE   C. TRUE   D. TRUE   E. FALSE

A 10 bit computer contains: - 2 10 grey scale levels = 1024

As the eye can only detect such a limited number of grey scales, the importance of 'windowing ' becomes apparent.

Background subtraction = subtracting the same number from each of the pixel values thus increasing contrast

Frame averaging is sometimes called temporal filtering

Noise reduction is achieved by low pass spatial filtering whilst edge enhancement is achieved by high pass spatial filtering

Ref: Farr & Allisy-Roberts. Physics for Medical Imaging. 1st Edition. W B Saunders Co Ltd.

ANSWER 12
A. FALSE   B. TRUE   C. FALSE   D. TRUE   E. FALSE

The sensitivity and field of view of a parallel hole collimator remain the same at distance

A convergent collimator would magnify an image

Pinhole collimators are used for imaging small superficial organs eg thyroid

With both convergent and divergent collimators, the back of an organ is magnified differently compared to the front. This leads to geometric distortion

Ref: Farr & Allisy-Roberts. Physics for Medical Imaging. 1st Edition. W B Saunders Co Ltd.

ANSWER 13
A. TRUE   B. FALSE   C. TRUE   D. FALSE   E. TRUE

The spatial resolution in SPECT = 15mm; PET = 5mm

Attenuation correction is applied pre-processing

Ref: Farr & Allisy-Roberts. Physics for Medical Imaging. 1st Edition. W B Saunders Co Ltd.

ANSWER 14
A. TRUE   B. TRUE   C. FALSE   D. FALSE   E. TRUE

Breast: Wt 0.05

Lung: Wt 0.12

Ref: Farr & Allisy-Roberts. Physics for Medical Imaging. 1st Edition. W B Saunders Co Ltd.

ANSWER 15

A. TRUE   B. TRUE   C. FALSE   D. TRUE   E. FALSE

With film badges, it is possible to identify the type and energy of an exposure due to the presence of the double coated emulsion and the various filters in the badge itself

TLDs are affective over a very wide range of doses (0.1-2,000 mSv)

Ref: Farr & Allisy-Roberts. Physics for Medical Imaging. 1st Edition. W B Saunders Co Ltd.

ANSWER 16

A. TRUE   B. TRUE   C. TRUE   D. TRUE   E. FALSE

Sound is attenuated exponentially with depth of travel

Ref: Farr & Allisy-Roberts. Physics for Medical Imaging. 1st Edition. W B Saunders Co Ltd.

ANSWER 17

A. TRUE   B. FALSE   C. TRUE   D. TRUE   E. TRUE

Flow away from the transducer is usually manifest as the colour blue. However the operator may reverse this setting at the console.

Ref: Farr & Allisy-Roberts. Physics for Medical Imaging. 1st Edition. W B Saunders Co Ltd.

ANSWER 18

A. FALSE   B. FALSE   C. FALSE   D. FALSE   E. TRUE

Water and CSF appear bright on T2 weighted imaging

Proton density weighted imaging; long TR:1,000-3,000 ms

Proton density weighted images tend to produce greater signal and less noise, and therefore high signal to noise ratio

Image contrast is principally due to differences in the proton density of the tissues

Indeed most tissues having a high proton density appear bright on proton density weighted imaging

Ref: Farr & Allisy-Roberts. Physics for Medical Imaging. 1st Edition. W B Saunders Co Ltd.

ANSWER 19

A. TRUE   B. TRUE   C. FALSE   D. TRUE   E. TRUE

Increasing the tip angle increases signal

Decreasing the band width of the receiver decreases noise, by picking up less of the spectrum of noise frequencies

Decreasing slice thickness decreases signal by reducing voxel size

Spin echo generally gives a bigger signal than in GRE

The use of surface coils decrease noise

Ref: Farr & Allisy-Roberts. Physics for Medical Imaging. 1st Edition. W B Saunders Co Ltd.

ANSWER 20
A. TRUE   B. TRUE   C. TRUE   D. FALSE   E. FALSE

The housing and supporting plates of an xray image intensifier should provide shielding equivalent to at least 2mm lead for 100 kV. From 100-150 kV an additional lead equivalent of 0.01mm per kV is required. The lead equivalence should be clearly stated on the equipment.

In mammography the total permanent filtration should never be less than 0.03mm molybdenum (equivalent to 0.5mm aluminium).

Ref: AC1/185, AC2/7, AC1/184, AC2/12: IRR 88.

ANSWER 21
A. TRUE   B. TRUE   C. TRUE   D. FALSE   E. FALSE

Though the primary fissure divides the superior surface the deepest fissure is the horizontal fissure

A CT of the upper cerebellum contains the cerebellum anteriorly and the occipital lobes posterolaterally. This is because the superior surface of cerebellum slopes upwards from posterior to anterior.

Refs:
Anatomy for Diagnostic Imaging. Ryan & McNicholas. W B Saunders Co Ltd.
Essential Anatomy by Lumley, Craven & Aitken. 3rd Edition. Churchill Livingstone.
Clinical Anatomy by Harold Ellis. 8th Edition. Churchill Livingstone.

ANSWER 22
A. FALSE   B. FALSE   C. TRUE   D. TRUE   E. TRUE

The calcaneum is the largest tarsal bone

Ossification of the talus begins in the 7th fetal month

Refs:
Last's Anatomy. McMinn. 9th Edition. Churchill Livingstone.
Gray's Anatomy. 38th Edition. Churchill Livingstone.

ANSWER 23
A. FALSE   B. FALSE   C. FALSE   D. FALSE   E. TRUE

The posterior cruciate is attached to the medial femoral condyle

The anterior cruciate prevents anterior displacement of the tibia

The semimembranosus bursa may communicate indirectly with the knee joint via the gastrocnemius bursa

Cruciate ligaments are of very low signal on T1 weighted MRI scans

Refs:
Last's Anatomy. McMinn. 9th Edition. Churchill Livingstone.
Anatomy for Diagnostic Imaging. Ryan & McNicholas. W B Saunders Co Ltd.

ANSWER 24

A. FALSE   B. TRUE   C. TRUE   D. TRUE   E. TRUE

Four views are used if scaphoid injury is suspected

Refs:
Anatomy for Diagnostic Imaging. Ryan & McNicholas. W B Saunders Co Ltd.
Diagnostic Radiography. Bryan. 3rd Edition. Churchill Livingstone.
An Atlas of Anatomy Basic to Radiology. Meschan. W B Saunders Co Ltd.

ANSWER 25

A. TRUE   B. TRUE   C. TRUE   D. FALSE   E. FALSE

The radial nerve lies dorso-lateral to the humerus

The brachial artery lies medial to the humerus on brachialis and the triceps muscles

Refs:
Last's Anatomy. McMinn. 9th Edition. Churchill Livingstone.
Gray's Anatomy. 38th Edition. Churchill Livingstone.

ANSWER 26

A. TRUE   B. TRUE   C. FALSE   D. TRUE   E. FALSE

The obturator artery passes above the obturator membrane

Coccygeus lies below piriformis

Refs:
Last's Anatomy. McMinn. 9th Edition. Churchill Livingstone.
Gray's Anatomy. 38th Edition. Churchill Livingstone.

ANSWER 27

A. FALSE   B. TRUE   C. TRUE   D. TRUE   E. FALSE

The ovaries are supplied by the ovarian artery directly from the aorta

The ovary attaches to the uterus by the suspensory ligament of the ovary

Refs:
Last's Anatomy. McMinn. 9th Edition. Churchill Livingstone.
Anatomy for Diagnostic Imaging. Ryan & McNicholas. W B Saunders Co Ltd.

ANSWER 28

A. FALSE   B. TRUE   C. TRUE   D. TRUE   E. FALSE

The abdominal aorta commences at T12

The inferior epigastric arteries are branches of the external iliac arteries

Refs:
Last's Anatomy. McMinn. 9th Edition. Churchill Livingstone.
Anatomy for Diagnostic Imaging. Ryan & McNicholas. W B Saunders Co Ltd.

ANSWER 29
A. TRUE   B. FALSE   C. TRUE   D. FALSE   E. TRUE

The GB is absent in 0.05% of cases

The GB is double in 0.025% of cases

Refs:
Last's Anatomy. McMinn. 9th Edition. Churchill Livingstone.
Anatomy for Diagnostic Imaging. Ryan & McNicholas. W B Saunders Co Ltd.

ANSWER 30
A. TRUE   B. TRUE   C. FALSE   D. FALSE   E. TRUE

The bare area of the liver drains to para-aortic nodes

The inferior surface of the diaphragm drains to para-aortic nodes

Refs:
Last's Anatomy. McMinn. 9th Edition. Churchill Livingstone.
Gray's Anatomy. 38th Edition. Churchill Livingstone.

ANSWER 31
A. TRUE   B. TRUE   C. FALSE   D. TRUE   E. TRUE

The Inferior epigastric veins drain into the external iliac veins

Ref: Last's Anatomy. McMinn. 9th Edition. Churchill Livingstone.

ANSWER 32
A. FALSE   B. FALSE   C. TRUE   D. TRUE   E. TRUE

There are 7 TRUE, 3 FALSE and 2 floating pairs of ribs.

Each typical rib articulates with the same vertebral level and the one above it.

Refs:
Anatomy for Diagnostic Imaging. Ryan & McNicholas. W B Saunders Co Ltd.
Essential Anatomy by Lumley, Craven & Aitken. 3rd Edition. Churchill Livingstone.
Clinical Anatomy by Harold Ellis. 8th Edition. Churchill Livingstone.

ANSWER 33
A. FALSE   B. TRUE   C. FALSE   D. TRUE   E. TRUE

It's the posterior wall which is smooth into which the great vein drains.

The fossa ovalis lies at the lower part of the inter-atrial septum.

Refs:
Anatomy for Diagnostic Imaging. Ryan & McNicholas. W B Saunders Co Ltd.
Essential Anatomy by Lumley, Craven & Aitken. 3rd Edition. Churchill Livingstone.
Clinical Anatomy by Harold Ellis. 8th Edition. Churchill Livingstone.

ANSWER 34

A. TRUE   B. FALSE   C. TRUE   D. FALSE   E. FALSE

Thoracic duct pierces the diaphragm at T12.

The right lymphatic duct is only 1cm long.

The normal length of thoracic duct is 45cm.

Refs:
Anatomy for Diagnostic Imaging. Ryan & McNicholas. W B Saunders Co Ltd.
Essential Anatomy by Lumley,Craven & Aitken. 3rd Edition. Churchill Livingstone.
Clinical Anatomy by Harold Ellis. 8th Edition. Churchill Livingstone.

ANSWER 35

A. TRUE   B. FALSE   C. TRUE   D. FALSE   E. FALSE

The vocal cords lie superior to the cricothyroid membrane

The true vocal cords are abducted during gentle respiration

The epiglottis does not calcify

Refs:
Anatomy for Diagnostic Imaging. Ryan & McNicholas. W B Saunders Co Ltd.
Essential Anatomy by Lumley,Craven & Aitken. 3rd Edition. Churchill Livingstone.
Clinical Anatomy by Harold Ellis. 8th Edition. Churchill Livingstone.

ANSWER 36

A. FALSE   B. FALSE   C. FALSE   D. FALSE   E. FALSE

Sternocleidomastoid has one head attached to the medial one third of the clavicle

Scalenus anterior is attached to C3-C6

The phrenic nerve lies anterior to the scalenus anterior

Scalenus medius is attached to the first rib

There are only four pairs of strap muscles anteriorly. These are sternothyroid, sternohyoid, omohyoid and thyrohyoid

Refs:
Anatomy for Diagnostic Imaging. Ryan & McNicholas. W B Saunders Co Ltd.
Essential Anatomy by Lumley,Craven & Aitken. 3rd Edition. Churchill Livingstone.
Clinical Anatomy by Harold Ellis. 8th Edition. Churchill Livingstone.

ANSWER 37

A. FALSE   B. TRUE   C. FALSE   D. TRUE   E. TRUE

The third cranial nerve has only motor and para-sympathetic motor fibres

The fourth cranial nerve enters the orbit through the superior orbital fissure

Refs:
Anatomy for Diagnostic Imaging. Ryan & McNicholas. W B Saunders Co Ltd.

Essential Anatomy by Lumley,Craven & Aitken. 3rd Edition. Churchill Livingstone.
Clinical Anatomy by Harold Ellis. 8th Edition. Churchill Livingstone.

ANSWER 38
A. FALSE   B. TRUE   C. FALSE   D. FALSE   E. TRUE

The ascending aorta is only 5cm long

The right main bronchus lies posterior to the ascending aorta

The left vagus nerve is posterior to the aorta however the phrenic nerve lies anterior to it

Refs:
Anatomy for Diagnostic Imaging. Ryan & McNicholas. W B Saunders Co Ltd.
Essential Anatomy by Lumley,Craven & Aitken. 3rd Edition. Churchill Livingstone.
Clinical Anatomy by Harold Ellis. 8th Edition. Churchill Livingstone.

ANSWER 39
A. TRUE   B. TRUE   C. TRUE   D. TRUE   E. FALSE

Tympanic antrum arises from the endoderm

Refs:
Anatomy for Diagnostic Imaging. Ryan & McNicholas. W B Saunders Co Ltd.
Essential Anatomy by Lumley,Craven & Aitken. 3rd Edition. Churchill Livingstone.
Clinical Anatomy by Harold Ellis. 8th Edition. Churchill Livingstone.

ANSWER 40
A. TRUE   B. TRUE   C. TRUE   D. TRUE   E. FALSE

Mandible arises from the first pharyngeal arch (Meckels cartilage)

Refs:
Anatomy for Diagnostic Imaging. Ryan & McNicholas. W B Saunders Co Ltd.
Essential Anatomy by Lumley,Craven & Aitken. 3rd Edition. Churchill Livingstone.
Clinical Anatomy by Harold Ellis. 8th Edition. Churchill Livingstone.

ANSWER 41
A. TRUE   B. TRUE   C. FALSE   D. FALSE   E. FALSE

An ascending urethrogram demonstrates up to the distal or external sphinctre. The Foley catheter balloon lies in the fossa navicularis. Paediatric bladder volumes increase by 30 mls per annum.

Ref: Grainger & Allison. Diagnostic Radiology. 3rd Edition. Churchill Livingstone.

ANSWER 42
A. TRUE   B. FALSE   C. TRUE   D. FALSE   E. TRUE

The renal cortex is thicker laterally rather than medially. The thickness between the capsule and the margin of the sinus echoes is the definition of parenchymal thickness.

Ref: Grainger & Allison. Diagnostic Radiology. 3rd Edition. Churchill Livingstone.

ANSWER 43
A. TRUE   B. FALSE   C. FALSE   D. TRUE   E. TRUE

The dose of a direct radionuclide study is 20 times less tha a radiographis one. Technique of choice in young girls for investigating UTI's, and in the follow up of known cases of vesicoureteric refluxations. This technique requires catheterisation. A direct micturating cystogram is at least as sensitive at detecting reflux as the radiographic technique.

Ref: Grainger & Allison. Diagnostic Radiology. 3rd Edition. Churchill Livingstone.

ANSWER 44
A. TRUE   B. TRUE   C. FALSE   D. FALSE   E. TRUE

Other causes of failure to opacify the gallbladder should be excluded first including malabsorbtion, hepatic failure and failure to take the pills. A preliminary film is not mandatory however this is controversial, some authors suggesting that up to 6% of calculi are missed without this film.

Ref: Whitehouse & Worthington. Techniques in Diagnostic Imaging. 3rd Edition. Blackwell Science Ltd.

ANSWER 45
A. FALSE   B. TRUE   C. TRUE   D. FALSE   E. FALSE

Following cholecystectomy the CBD can measure up to 10 mm. The upper limit of normal for the pancreatic duct is 2.5 mm. Intraductal transducers have frequencies of 20-30 MHz.

Ref: Grainger & Allison. Diagnostic Radiology. 3rd Edition. Churchill Livingstone.

ANSWER 46
A. TRUE   B. TRUE   C. FALSE   D. FALSE   E. TRUE

A transvenous large cutting needle biopsy is the method of choice in severe clotting disorders. A percutaneous biopsy tract can be embolised percutaneously with coils or gel.

Ref: Grainger & Allison. A Guide to Radiological Procedures. 3rd Edition. W B Saunders Co Ltd.

ANSWER 47
A. TRUE   B. FALSE   C. TRUE   D. TRUE   E. TRUE

The pancreas has a purely arterial blood supply.

Ref: Grainger & Allison. Diagnostic Radiology. 3rd Edition. Churchill Livingstone.

ANSWER 48
A. FALSE   B. TRUE   C. TRUE   D. TRUE   E. FALSE

The film cassette and tube move together around the centre point in opposite directions. In addition at the same time the film cassette which is curved rotates around its own axis to allow the film to be exposed by a collimated beam from one end to the other during exposure. The arc may be eliptical to simulate the shape of the dental arches.

Ref: Bell and Finlay. Basic Radiographic Positioning and Anatomy. 1st Edition. Bailliere Tindall.

ANSWER 49

A. TRUE   B. FALSE   C. FALSE   D. FALSE   E. FALSE

Cine has higher frame rates than rapid serial roll film. Dynamic studies should only be performed if a motility disorder is suspected or to define pharyngo-oesophageal junctional anatomy. 6 - 16 frames per second

are required. Single boluses are followed as motor activity is affects by second bolus.

Ref: Whitehouse & Worthington. Techniques in Diagnostic Imaging. 3rd Edition. Blackwell Science Ltd.

ANSWER 50

A. FALSE   B. FALSE   C. TRUE   D. FALSE   E. TRUE

Endoscopic ultrasound is performed busing an oblique view linear array probe. The patient lies on their left side.

Ref: Whitehouse & Worthington. Techniques in Diagnostic Imaging. 3rd Edition. Blackwell Science Ltd.

ANSWER 51

A. FALSE   B. TRUE   C. TRUE   D. TRUE   E. FALSE

Barium is run in in the left lateral position or prone. The transverse colon should be two-thirds full before contrast is drained out. Turning the patient twice theorectically it gives more even coating. Air insufflation in the supine position will cause overspill of contrast into terminal ileum as ileocaecal valve is posterolateral. Therefore insufflation of air should be in the prone position.

Ref: Whitehouse & Worthington. Techniques in Diagnostic Imaging. 3rd Edition. Blackwell Science Ltd.

ANSWER 52

A. TRUE   B. TRUE   C. FALSE   D. TRUE   E. TRUE

The milk feed is divided into two parts. Tracer is added to one part which is given first. The infant is placed supine or prone. Dynamic imaging is only required if aspiration is suspected.

Ref: Chapman & Nakielny. A Guide to Radiological Procedures. 3rd Edition. W B Saunders Co Ltd.

ANSWER 53

A. TRUE   B. FALSE   C. TRUE   D. FALSE   E. TRUE

The diameter of guide wires in measured in inches. A standard paediatric wire is 0.025".

Ref: Whitehouse & Worthington. Techniques in Diagnostic Imaging. 3rd Edition. Blackwell Science Ltd.

ANSWER 54
A. TRUE   B. TRUE   C. FALSE   D. FALSE   E. FALSE

IV DSA requires 350 - 370 mg per ml instead of 240 mg per ml of contrast. Intravenous ionic contrast injections have twice as many contrast reactions as intra-arterial. An antecubital approach can be used. Only with patients with a cardiac history need cardiac monitoring.

Ref: Chapman & Nakielny. A Guide to Radiological Procedures. 3rd Edition. W B Saunders Co Ltd.

ANSWER 55
A. FALSE   B. FALSE   C. FALSE   D. TRUE   E. FALSE

Sagittal obliques are planned along the plane of the ACL. Sagittal volume sequence are perfemed again to visualise the ACL. Only in patients with specific symptoms such as anterior knee pain are axial sequences required. Each knee requires a separate coil.

Ref: MRI in Orthopaedics and Sports Medicine. Stoller. Lippincott Raven.

ANSWER 56
A. TRUE   B. FALSE   C. TRUE   D. FALSE   E. TRUE

Wrist arthrograms are only performed in single contrast. The injection is into the radiocarpal compartment. Early views are requied to detect leakage into the midcarpal joint.

Ref: Chapman & Nakielny. A Guide to Radiological Procedures. 3rd Edition. W B Saunders Co Ltd.

ANSWER 57
A. FALSE   B. TRUE   C. TRUE   D. FALSE   E. FALSE

Pulmonary angiography is contraindicated if the mean PA pressure is greater than 50 mm per Hg. A vascular sheath is not necessary. It is the femoral vein that is punctured for this procedure !

Ref: Chapman & Nakielny. A Guide to Radiological Procedures. 3rd Edition. W B Saunders Co Ltd.

ANSWER 58
A. FALSE   B. TRUE   C. FALSE   D. TRUE   E. TRUE

10-100 micrometer particles are used. Technegas contains carbon particles and is used in ventilation studies. Less than 0.5% of total capillary bed is occluded.

Ref: Chapman & Nakielny. A Guide to Radiological Procedures. 3rd Edition. W B Saunders Co Ltd.

ANSWER 59

A. TRUE   B. FALSE   C. TRUE   D. FALSE   E. FALSE

Patients must be able to lie supine or semi recumbant during perfusion study. Right to left cardiac shunt is a contraindication. Less than 0.5% of capillary bed is occluded, so pulmonary hypertension must be severe to be a contraindication. The injection is intravenous through a peripheral vein.

Ref: Chapman & Nakielny. A Guide to Radiological Procedures. 3rd Edition. W B Saunders Co Ltd.

ANSWER 60

A. FALSE   B. TRUE   C. FALSE   D. TRUE   E. TRUE

The windows should range from be centered around 275. Both a narrow window width of 700 and a wide window width of up to 1600 are used. The dose from a 1mm section is the same as that from a 2mm section because the beam that passes through the patient and is then collimated to the selective thickness. Expiration scans are helpful to look for airtrapping in a selected population.

Ref: Grainger & Allison. Diagnostic Radiology. 3rd Edition. Churchill Livingstone.

QBase Radiology on CD-ROM

SYSTEM REQUIREMENTS

An IBM compatible PC with a mimimum 80386 processor and 4mb of RAM

VGA Monitor set up to display at least 256 colours

CD-ROM drive

Windows 3.1 or higher with Microsoft compatible mouse

INSTALLATION INSTRUCTIONS

The program will install the appropriate files onto your hard drive. It requires the QBase CD-ROM to be installed in the D:\drive.

In order to run QBase the CD-ROM must be in the drive.

Print Readme.txt and Helpfile.txt on the CD-ROM for fuller instructions and user manual

WINDOWS 95/98/2000

1. Insert the QBase CD-ROM into the drive **D:**
2. From the **Start Menu**, select the **Run option**
3. Type **D:\setup.exe** and press enter or return
4. **Follow the Full Installation** option and accept the default directory for installation of QBase.
   The installation program creates a folder called **QBase** containing the program icon and another called Exams into which you can save previous exam attempts.
5. To run QBase double click the **QBase** icon in the Qbase folder. From Windows Explorer double click the **QBase.exe** file in the QBase folder.

WINDOWS 3.1/WINDOWS FOR WORKGROUPS 3.11

1. Insert the QBase CD-ROM into the drive **D:**
2. From the **File Menu**, selct the **RUN option**
3. Type **D:\setup.exe** and press enter or return
4. Follow the instructions given by the installation program. Select the **Full Installation** option and accept the default directory for installation of QBase
   The installation program creates a program window and directory called **QBase** containing the program icon. It also creates a directory called Exams into which you can save previous attempts.
5. To run QBase click on the **QBase** icon in the QBase program. From File Manager double click the **QBase.exe** file in the QBase directory

NOTES

NOTES

NOTES

NOTES

NOTES

NOTES